At a S'
by Harold La....

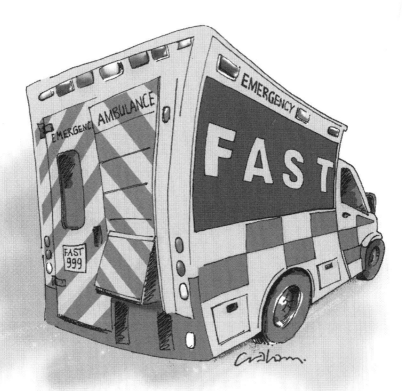

Book designed and illustrated by Graham Wilkins
Illustrations©Graham Wilkins
www.grahamwilkins.design

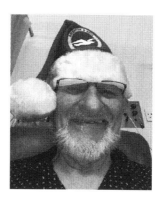

To those who know him, Harold had always been prone to accepting challenges head-on. Whether it was walking 640 miles along the South West Coastal Path with Fargo, a puppet frog, attached to his boots and rucksack; Climbing the three Highest Peaks in England, Scotland and Wales within 24 hours; Picking up a pebble from the Irish sea, then walking across England before throwing it in to the North sea; organising a 'Yeti Hunt' which involved walking the West Highland Way from Glasgow to Fort William, before scaling Ben Nevis.

It was no surprise to anybody, then, that when he suffered a stroke, he found it interesting enough to keep notes throughout his treatment.

'At a Stroke - a Stroke Survivor's Journey' gives a rare insight, from a patient's perspective, into the trials, tribulations and humour, associated with Stroke recovery, and is the culmination of his scribbling.

Besides promising to write a number of books that he has been procrastinating about over the past 20 years, he is now kept busy speaking to groups, schools and organisations about stroke awareness and of course getting the message across in his own inimitable and humorous style.

For purchase and further information vist the website:
www.atastroke.co.uk

Acknowledgements

I would like to express my sincere thanks to the following for their invaluable assistance during the writing of 'At a Stroke'. Their encouragement and most importantly, their critiques were a massive help to me.

My good friends, Mike and Sandy Fagg; Ralph Burton; Geoff Lee; Steve Booth; Robin Barnett and John Dowling, who were all prepared to give up their time, at my request, to read the manuscript. I would like to thank Diana Collis at Jericho Writers, who was given the task of editing and appraising my work, for her honest and constructive feedback.

Thank you, Keith Pike and the 'A team' at the Talking Newspaper Association for allowing me to read extracts from my book to the listeners. I hope you haven't lost any!

Thanks to my friends at the Writers' Group for also indulging me and listening politely to extracts, without a hint of a yawn. I appreciated their genuine encouragement.

A huge thank you to my friends Steve Booth and Graham Wilkins. Both provided the technical skills required to publish 'At a Stroke' to a highly professional standard. I also consider myself to be a very lucky bloke to have had Graham, a talented artist and designer, agree to illustrate the book.

'At a Stroke' is a memoir, though not a strict diary of events. The characters are representative of the wonderful people who were part of my story, but any resemblance to specific individuals is purely co-incidental.

Harold Lawrence

A donation will be made to the Stroke Association from the proceeds of each sale of 'At a Stroke'

Foreword

A stroke is everyone's worst nightmare. Order, routine, holiday plans, Christmas – all the cherished and under-appreciated joys of normality are replaced in an instant with disorder and confusion, dizzying disorientation, disability and terror.

For any stroke victim the twin options are stark. Go under or fight back. It is typical of the man that there was only one choice for Harold Lawrence.

As consultants muttered in disconcerting huddles and in the MRI scanner's claustrophobic closeness road drills pounded his brain Harold, writer and fighter, turned not to self-pity but to a notebook. Who else would have the presence of mind to keep a record as a succession of bewildering misfortunes overtook him?

The result is At a Stroke, a remarkable work by any calculation. It is a telling insight into the post-stroke experience, one that will undoubtedly be of invaluable service and comfort to others confronted with the same challenges.

More than that, with a clarity which is remarkable given the circumstances, it is acute and objective observation of the NHS at work – polyglot yet endearingly unified - one that, despite his own urgent needs at the time, reveals Harold's compassion for his fellow human beings.

Even more remarkably, his sense of humour did not desert him in his hour of need and the irony of his circumstances and those of a rich tapestry of fellow-travellers twinkles amid the trauma.

John Dowling
Author and Journalist

This Book is dedicated to Carers everywhere and especially to my dear wife, Angela; the wonderful staff of the NHS, including the members of the Community team; my fellow Stroke survivors. Without the encouragement, guidance and inspiration of all these people, it is doubtful that this book would ever have been written.

I love you all.

Prologue

"Wake up! It's 2017. Happy New Year!"

The year had started for me when Angela woke me up from a deep sleep.

On the TV, the screen was filled by the spectacle of thousands of pounds worth of fireworks, gyrating, cavorting and bursting across the London sky in a kaleidoscope of many colours. Each explosion ecstatically cheered on by thousands of revellers. Over the years, I too have similarly celebrated and have collected memories of popping champagne corks and other revelries, but now I am much more attracted to 'a quiet night in'.

Perhaps, if I had known what surprises the year had in store for me, it would have been wiser to have continued snoozing, and allow it to carry on without me.

I like to think of myself as a pragmatist. I sincerely believe that there is no option other than to manage the cards as they are dealt, though, at that moment I didn't know the 2017 pack contained so many jokers. From my perspective, it was to become a year like no other on this earth. It was scary.

Like many other people, I was overwhelmed and bored by the apparent surfeit of fake news and the never-ending flow of 'doom and gloom' fed daily via the media. Globally, it seemed, toxic rhetoric by the likes of Trump, Putin and Kim Jong Un threatened the world with imminent annihilation, whilst politicians in the UK were diverted from establishing compassionate policies and the protection of vital services by the time-consuming and seemingly impossible 'Brexit' dilemma. Could it get any worse? It could and it did!

With the year still in its infancy, I was, despite, to my knowledge, being symptom-free, diagnosed to have bowel cancer and in July I had to undergo an operation to remove part of my colon. I, fortunately recovered well, and I was, after this temporary interruption, soon back on my merry way, until November, when

I was once again unexpectedly stopped in my tracks by a kidney stone that left me in considerable pain and kicking my heels at the A&E Department of my local Hospital.

"Enough is enough" I had thought. "I don't want another year like this, I'm glad it is nearly over!"

But nothing is over 'til the Matron sings!

Chapter 1

I was propped up on four pillows in a ward of the District Hospital, where I had ended up, totally unexpectedly, after suffering a suspected stroke, in the early hours, of a December morning.

Harold Lawrence, has had a stroke? Impossible! This is the sort of thing that sadly happens to other people, but not to him.

Barely twenty-four hours earlier, not unlike millions of other people, I had been up to my eyes in, what was to me, normal 'day to day' activities. As usual, it was me racing against the clock. Why does it seem that there are never enough hours in the day? I had a seventy-mile round trip to Brighton in order to pick up some Christmas presents for my grandsons; pay a balance owed to the Travel Agent for the pre-booked 'Northern Lights Experience'; and confirm arrangements with the Community Manager at the local Tesco store for a charity collection to be held later in the week.

I went to bed, with my head full of plans that would carry me through tomorrow. At lunchtime I was due to speak to the Rotary Club about the progress of the Schools' Young Writers Competition, as well as seeking volunteers to be placed on the rota for 'tin rattling' duties outside of the store.

Then, I remembered that I had planned to write some important letters to local dignitaries, inviting them to be guests at the AGM and Presentation Event of the disability football team that I had founded fifteen years ago. I had the AGM agenda to prepare in addition to the programme for the Presentations. I also had to put the final touches to the annual Club Magazine before sending it off to the printers! I had a lot to do, and it was important that I caught the last post. After all, post, at this time of the year, can be delayed in the Christmas rush.

I had a myriad of tasks to complete before the Christmas Holiday.

There was so much on my mind that, although I was tired, I was having one of those nights when dropping off to sleep seemed a step too far and I was trying to come to terms with a restless and seemingly endless night.

At approximately 3.00 a.m. I felt a sharp pain in my neck and the bed seemed to rock. I concluded that I must have slept awkwardly and had momentarily trapped a nerve. Now wide awake, I decided to have a natural break, not an unusual nocturnal activity for a bloke in his seventies, and tip-tapped my way through the darkness towards the bathroom door. Suddenly the bedroom revolved like a washing machine with me as its contents. The wardrobe flew past my eyes a couple of times (goodness knows how that got into the machine!), as I seemed to be whisked around before being dumped on the floor. I dug my fingernails in to the carpet as a precaution against the risk of ending up on the ceiling. Like the proverbial drunk found face down across the pavement with his fingers clinging to the kerb, I shouted "Help me, I can't hang on much longer!"

Angela, her sleep disturbed by the commotion, was not over-impressed with my instant, self-diagnosis that I was only suffering from a touch of vertigo. I somehow managed to crawl back in to bed, but I soon discovered it was impossible for me to balance in a sitting position. Angela, having recovered from the initial shock, and now fully conscious, proved the wisdom of the old saying that the spectator sees most of the game. Apparently, the colour had gone from my cheeks and there was a blue tinge around my mouth. I certainly felt very cold, yet I was sweating profusely, and to all intent and purpose, I might just as well have stepped from under the shower, as my pyjamas were wringing wet. Despite this frightening turn-of-events of which we were both trying to make sense and deal with, Angela calmly assumed control and dialled 999.

After what seemed an age, but in fact was quite a short time, an ambulance arrived. Two paramedics greeted me cheerfully as they followed Angela into the bedroom. They asked me a couple of questions about the circumstances of my collapse, tested my blood pressure, took my temperature. It seemed to take them no time at all to decide that the symptoms I was presenting could possibly signify that I may have had a stroke. I was certainly feeling strange and trying to sit up and balance was still an issue, but, a stroke? They've got to be wrong! The very word 'STROKE' caused shockwaves to reverberate through my body.

After Angela provided me with a pair of perspiration-free pyjamas and matching dressing-gown, the paramedics strapped me into a wheelchair, and with some difficulty, man-handled it, together with its 96.56kg occupant (that's 15st. 3 lb in old money), up a flight of stairs before loading me into the back of their vehicle.

My night was becoming curiouser and curiouser, unmatched to any in my whole life. One minute I was tossing and turning in bed, the next minute tossing and turning in a washing machine, and now swaying on a stretcher to the rhythm of the ambulance as it hurtled along the road, with its flashing blue lights reflecting off the rain-washed surface.

The paramedic checked my blood pressure and temperature, probably two or three times during the journey whilst complimenting me on my choice of pyjamas and dressing gown. "They're smart, where did you buy 'em?" he said, "When I come off shift, I'm going to M&S's and buy a set for myself".
It was a conversation, though surreal, that was, under the circumstances, ordinary enough to reduce the drama of suddenly and unexpectedly rushing through the night in the back of an ambulance with blue lights flashing to nothing more than an adventure or weird dream.

I was received into the A&E Department at the District General Hospital and greeted by a team exuding efficiency laced with smiles. Observations were recorded of my blood pressure, sugar levels and temperature. Being new to the experience, I was unaware that "obs", as this procedure is referred to by the medical staff, would become the routine for a minimum of four times a day for the next month of my life. There was some concern that my core temperature was well below normal and I was provided with a duvet that had hot air blown under it from some sort of generator contraption. It was pure luxury, and not once did the nursing staff communicate any concerns to me, though, according to Angela, my condition was causing a degree of anxiety. In fact, they were quite complicit in humouring me when I pretended that I was impatient to receive any other spa treatments that might be available!

Everybody was extremely busy, yet at that moment I was grateful to be at the centre of their world. I suppose that at such a time of confusion and fear every patient places their needs above that of others. I guess it is selfish, but only human. A doctor came to examine me. It appeared that he had been called from his bed. His hair lacked a comb and I noticed the sleeves of his pyjamas poking from under the cuffs of his crumpled jacket. (I am not so sure that the paramedic would have coveted the Doc's nightwear with the same enthusiasm that he showed towards mine).

A stethoscope was applied to my heart and lungs and I was then wheeled off to the X-ray department to have a scan. My only memory of this was that I suddenly vomited! The nurse, who was accompanying me, seemed totally unphased and said, as she cleaned-up me and the trolley, that I might have banged my head when I had collapsed and that I was probably suffering from concussion. Though this was never again mentioned, it is more than likely that I had banged my head, and as I have already said, the scanning process was completely blanked from my mind, which might have been significant.

On my return to the A&E Department, the doctor told me that he had decided that I should be kept in for further tests and observations, and he had requested that a place be prepared for me in the acute stroke unit

I had been in A&E three hours by the time that all the initial 'obs' and scans had been completed. Night had become day when a hospital porter was eventually summoned to trundle the 'bed-ridden me' up to the Stroke ward.

On arrival, my bed was pushed into a bay which contained five other patients. I looked around me. None of my newly acquired neighbours looked too well compared to how I was feeling.

"I'll be home in a couple of days, Love" I said cheerily, as I waved farewell to a very tired and stressed looking Angela.

Chapter 2

Whilst settling into my new surroundings, I was asked to select what I wanted to eat from the lunch and supper menus, and as I had missed breakfast, I was also offered a slice of toast and marmalade together with a cup of tea. I sensed the merest hint of impatience shown by the enquirer at my hesitation before responding to these requests. It was still the middle of the night to me and I had found myself landed in a totally unfamiliar environment. I was still feeling confused by the speed of events and food was the least important thing on my mind. I had become a first former again in 'Big School'. Although I did not feel fear exactly, I seemed to lack confidence and felt unsure and discomforted as a new inmate within this institution to which I had unexpectedly been transported. I can only guess, but this must be how convicts feel when the iron gates clang shut behind them! Once I had been transferred to the hospital ward, it was as if I had strayed from my comfort zone, into the mystery land of C.S Lewis' Narnia. I recalled the 'washing machine' experience I had had earlier, and the sensation I had felt as the wardrobe seemed to flash past my prone body, and I was beginning to wonder whether I must have walked through it!

Everybody appeared to have a role and a rule. I reasoned that new patients, not unlike prisoners, need to learn quickly as the hospital routine is a well-tried system that works. Questions are politely brushed aside with platitudes such as, "Don't worry, we'll look after you; Doctor will be here, soon, and you can ask him; I'll have a word with Matron; Would you like some water? – we must keep you hydrated..." I soon understood that these caring people were assuming responsibility for the well-being and maintenance of my body. They are trained, practised, professionals that know what they are doing.

I have little understanding of matters medical and never harboured the ambition to learn, but I instinctively knew that I would need to adopt a coping strategy to make my stay in hospital a little easier.

At the risk of pretentiousness, but for what it's worth, I'm happy to share my strategy. We are all different and my coping mechanism is probably not infallible, but it worked for me. With a little bit of tweaking, it might well help others too. I pretended that I had been physically separated from my body! I then delivered it, like a vehicle in need of a service, into the hands of the 'medic-mechanics' to repair. I placed my complete trust in them, which is only right and not difficult to do. OK, mistakes happen, as they do in any well-ordered society, and these receive wide publicity. But the NHS also enjoys millions of successes that don't make the news.

Personally, I like to believe that the vast majority who join the medical profession are people that are driven by a desire to make the sick better. By adopting a positive attitude, patients can also become partners with the carers and help in the process of their own recovery.

Before long, I was visited by the Stroke specialist who was being trailed by a retinue of Registrar and medical students. (I thought there were only two visitors per bed allowed at any one time). He was a friendly man and introduced himself with a strong foreign accent. I did not catch the name, but I was sure that I would be able to find it out from one of the nurses. In the meantime, I decided that I would privately call him Doctor Egg, as at first sight, to me, he resembled one. I like to give people a name. It is only polite and helps to build on a relationship. I realised that if my private little joke leaked out, my theory could be seriously compromised, though I suspected that Doctor Egg might see the sunny side!

Doctor Egg referred to a file that had my name and patient number on the front cover. He discussed the contents with his student group and asked them a couple of, I presumed, pertinent questions. He averted his eyes to the floor, as he listened to their responses and nodded slowly, before focussing his attention back to me.

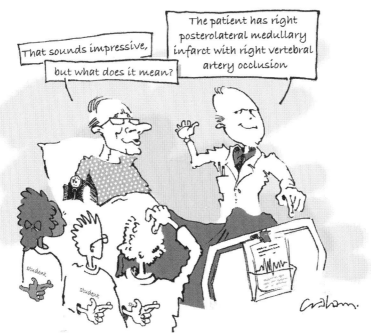

"Look up without moving your head" he instructed," look to the right, now to the left, squeeze my fingers with your right hand, now with your left hand. Hold your right arm up and now forwards, do the same with your left hand. You see my forefinger? I want you to touch the tip of this finger with your forefinger, now touch your nose. Thanks, now repeat, using the forefinger on your other hand, touch the tip of your nose and now the tip of my finger, good." I reckoned that I had accomplished all tasks satisfactory and was quietly pleased that his examination had proved easy and painless. He bowed his head in thought and after approximately ten seconds addressed the student gathering. "I would suggest that the patient has right posterolateral medullary infarct with right vertebral artery occlusion. I want him to have a CTD and an MRI."

As I have said, I have no medical pedigree. In fact, over the years I was always terrified by needles and medical procedures, not that I ever had anything other than the routine jabs, such as anti-diphtheria; tuberculosis; smallpox. I did once have a penicillin injection, to cure a boil, that made me faint. Pain wasn't the cause, only fear of the unknown!

"That sounds impressive," I said, desperately wishing to be one of the in crowd, "but what does it mean?"

He turned back to me. "Mr. Lawrence, you have definitely had a stroke, probably effecting part of the brain called the cerebellum in the region of the medulla oblongata. The cerebellum is the part of the brain which controls co-ordination and balance. Scans will be able to tell us more. You are doing very well, keep improving and you will be able to go home on Friday."

Without any further discussion, he and his coterie shuffled on to another bed and another patient, leaving me to quietly reflect on my situation.

I nodded my head and smiled, though none the wiser but pretending that I was now au fait with his diagnosis and at the same time pleased to receive the advice that I would be home by Friday.

I have had a Stroke. 'Stroke' is an emotive word and the event, itself, is undoubtedly life defining. If not fatal, metaphorically, it certainly brings the carousel to a shuddering halt.

How is it going to leave me? How will it alter mine and Angie's lives? Will we have to move to a more user-friendly house? Will I lose my independence? Will I have to give up driving? Will I ever stop feeling sorry for myself?

The immediate consequences were sobering. The planned holiday in Norway to see the Northern Lights, cancelled. Christmas Party with the Rotary Club and Christmas Lunch with the Writers' Group both cancelled. In fact, Christmas was odds on to being cancelled! But that's not all. I was halfway through organising the local schools' 'Young Writer' competition and that was left dangling. I would be unable to take my grandson to watch premiership football at Brighton. Everything, at least for the next few months, would seem to be out of bounds which included a planned trip to a West End Theatre. Yes, the negatives, initially, overwhelmed me. But, everything in life is a balance, and I found that a stream of positives began to flow through my mind and the perceived 'important' negatives started to diminish into insignificance.

Things that I had volunteered to do-when others had been reticent to take responsibility- I might have to give up. Perhaps the reticent others will have to be more forthcoming! I had to wait no longer than Angela's next visit to find out that other people had already assured her that they would take over, and that I was not to worry.

Neighbours, with whom Angela and I had only been on nodding terms, expressed their concern and sympathy as soon as they heard about my problem. Angela was immediately offered genuine support. She was besieged with offers of help. If she needed anything she only had to ask. It was wonderful to be reminded that there still exists generosity and kind heartedness within communities when the chips are down. We were profoundly touched and grateful. Clearly, I would never have put suffering a disabling attack–caused by an interruption of blood-flow to the brain-on my things to do list. But it was positive to learn that being the victim of a stroke could be an effective catalyst for turning acquaintances in to friends.

As the word spread wider about my unexpected infirmity, Angela was overwhelmed with many more offers of help and support. The telephone answer machine was soon full-up with messages wanting to know the situation, requests to visit, and love and support to all the family.

The postman was delivering handfuls of post. It was just like having a birthday, but even better, as the cards come in, day after day, and whilst some of the messages were very funny, others were quite profound. One person wrote, "Harold – the world needs you." It was not clear, however, whether he was referring to this world or the next.

It is unusual, I think, and a little bit unnerving, to learn what others think of you before the Grim Reaper calls. Obituaries and eulogies, I have noticed over the years, can often be somewhat exaggerated or spun in favour of the late departed. In fact, I have attended funerals that, when listening to the address, I have panicked, believing that I was attending the last rites of the wrong deceased.

One thing which really struck me, however, was the effect that the news of my Stroke had had as it reverberated around the town.

"Harold? No, it can't have happened to him!"

If it had this effect on friends and acquaintances, then one could only imagine how it was received by my nearest and dearest.

In the modern world, children, reach adulthood, leave the nest and forge lives independently from the nuclear family. It dawned on me how huge an impact my stroke must have had on the whole family. Mine were in shock. It was probably the first time that the kids had ever believed that their Dad's mortality was ever in question! Yes, it had caused them an immense amount of worry, yet it was the positivity of their love that sustained and supported me through this difficult time.

Throughout my life, I have been fortunate to enjoy good health. But the previous twelve months had resulted in me spending more time in the waiting rooms of hospitals, dentists and G.P.'s than over the three-quarters of a century of my previous existence. In fact, this pastime had become a major part of my social life. It is not difficult to fall into conversation with fellow patients, especially if reading 'retro-mags' such as 'National Geographic' or 'Horse and Hound' is not your bag! I have had some interesting chats, but inevitably the conversation centres around ailments and prescription drugs.

I am constantly amazed at ordinary folks' medical knowledge. I would hesitate to call these people party aninals, but I am convinced they would be an absolute boon to any pub quiz team.

One morning, I sat next to a woman who, unbeknown to me, was obviously keen to unburden her multifarious ailments on a willing listener. Naively, I gave her the opportunity.

"Hello!" I said, "lovely weather for the time of the year."

"Yes, it really cheers me up, but what with my ulcerated legs, diabetes, high blood-pressure, wonky heart and bad knees, I can't get out to enjoy it. It seems I spend most of my day taking various pills. Metformin, Lansoprazole, Apixaban, Cholecalciferol and Codeine for the pain. When I gets up in the morning, I rattle!" She gave a little laugh, "What pills do you take?"

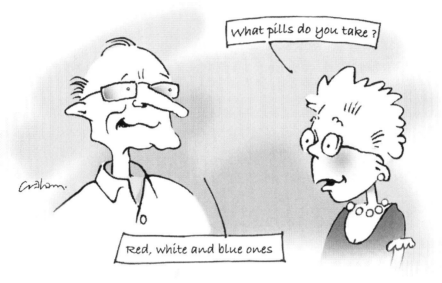

"Red, white and blue ones." I replied.

Though people, of a certain age, are often keen to discuss their medical problems with friends, as well as strangers, their own mortality is never, or extremely rarely, discussed. Stand-up comedians will sometimes irreverently joke about it, but it seems to me that the concept of death is still a difficult subject for a lot of people. I appreciate it is hardly an exciting prospect, but it is inevitable, and if it was included in general conversation along with the price of cheese, I am sure that it would greatly reduce the fear of the event if not the mystery.

The pressure of day to day living rarely affords the luxury of quiet moments in which to indulge in profound thought. So, as I had now found the time, I reckoned this had to be chalked up as another positive!

I looked around the ward. The patients to my right and left and opposite seemed to be very ill. I felt a bit of a fraud as, in my estimation, I was the fittest one there. It was almost embarrassing!

I was also astounded by the care and concern shown me by the hospital staff. Constantly checking my blood pressure and temperature whilst also looking after Angela's welfare and keeping her up to date with information on my condition. I quickly learned that carers are gold-dust and totally under-valued, that is until we desperately require their skills. They were devoting so much of their time to me when I knew that they were all so busy and their expertise constantly in demand from other patients. No one, it seems, fully appreciates the impact caring for stroke survivors must have on the carers.

The public are constantly being reminded by the medical profession, and through the media, that if we ignore the dangers of obesity, smoking, lack of exercise etc. we are in danger of having a stroke. A slight adjustment to lifestyle is probably all that is needed to keep healthy. But, when push comes to shove, such warnings go unheeded. According to statistics supplied by the Stroke Association, 100,000 people suffer a stroke in the UK every year.

I felt a sense of embarrassment at becoming one of the statistics, because I, too, had received those self-same warnings and failed to take them seriously. After all, I was OK and certainly enjoying my lifestyle.

An old saying came to my mind.

There's none so queer as folk 'cept me and thee. Yet even thee's a little queer!

Oh well, incorrigible that I obviously am, I've been lucky. After all, didn't the doctor say that, once all the tests have been completed, I'd be going home on Friday.

Chapter 3

It had been a long night. Sleep had been at a premium due to the constant toing and froing of the nursing staff, as they attended to the needs of patients and I was regularly disturbed, whenever I managed to doze off. I must have enjoyed some periods of sleep because the nurses always apologised for waking me in order to record my blood pressure, temperature and blood sugar readings or 'obs' as it is called. Why is it that nobody troubles you much about such things in the 'outside world,' yet within the institution it is a practice performed regularly, at least every four hours, and apparently holds body and soul together?

Earlier in the evening, before 'lights out', and feeling in need of the bathroom, I had attempted to get out of bed but was unable to stand even with help and became extremely dizzy. Strange really, because I still seemed fine. I was supplied with a cardboard jar in which to pee. I remember feeling rather self-conscious as it felt so undignified. Fortunately, these feelings of inhibition are merely a temporary problem as one acclimatises to 'in-patient culture'.

The nurses suggested that my blood pressure was too low and that for the time being I should remain resting in bed, and I was given a further three jars to see me through the night. By the morning, I had lined up the three cardboard jars of urine, neatly, beside my bed, like discarded shoes.

I've never understood what the numbers mean when blood pressure is taken. One of the nurses explained to me that blood pressure is measured in millimetres of mercury and is given in two figures. The first is systolic pressure and the second diastolic pressure. Still being none the wiser, I never-the-less nodded wisely and thanked her for the explanation. I made a mental note to read, if such a book exists, 'The Blood Pressure Guide for Dummies'.

The Housekeeping- staff appeared on the ward at approximately 6.00 am and, as usual, requested our preferences from the breakfast menu. Having been deprived of exercise and sleep, I had not gained any appetite. I also had a bit of a headache, but that was inevitable, I thought, after the upheaval of the past few hours. I had been told by a friend, who had spent time in the same hospital, some months earlier, that the food was rather unpalatable. Therefore, it was with little enthusiasm that I decided on a breakfast of porridge, marmalade on toast and orange juice. I am pleased to report that a well-prepared breakfast was served and despite my fears being stoked by the misinformation, I thoroughly enjoyed it!

I was temporarily off the nursing staff's radar, so I turned the bedside radio on to BBC Radio 4.

I'll catch up with the news on the 'Today' programme, I thought.

The headline story involved the NHS. Lord Kerslake had apparently resigned from the chairmanship of the Kings College Hospital Trust. He had stated that the government were refusing to understand and take on board the critical financial, staffing and resource shortages that the NHS was facing over the winter period.

When interviewed, he had said,

"... the dire NHS funding problems require a fundamental rethink of the way that the NHS is funded and organised..."

Mr. and Mrs. Average, at the start of the day, might well say "That's disgraceful, something should be done" before more personal and pressing business diverts them. They carry on with life and probably have little time to think about the matter any further. It is the sort of subject that might crop up in a conversation at the local pub, and there is bound to be a barrack room lawyer who simply resolves the problem in the time that it takes to sink a pint of best bitter.

BUT...

I was, no longer, 'Mr. Average Bloke'. I was occupying an NHS bed and if the noble Lord's statement truly reflected the reality of the situation, I was in the middle of a muddle. My present, as well as my future, was intrinsically integrated within the complexities of the problem.

As Lord Kerslake had concluded that his decision was clearly defined, based on his experience, I felt compelled to put my own mind in gear, too. What were my experiences and observations, so far, since this unexpected and seismic happening in my life? One thing was for sure, the workings of the NHS were now, not only relevant to me, but tangibly so.

The Ward was, without doubt, extremely busy.

Doctors, Nurses and Ancillary workers were compelled to work twelve-hour shifts. I was surrounded by personnel from a kaleidoscope of nations and cultures who, in common, treated each patient with care and kindness. It was noticeable that they managed critical situations with professionalism and good humour. To the layman, it seemed that their hard work and skills were sometimes treated with less respect than they deserved, by both management and some patients, which occasionally caused individuals moments of frustration and impacted on their morale. There may have been under-breath mutterings, but I feel certain that 'resignation' would have been a dirty word. I felt confident, based on my limited knowledge of the staff on the Stroke Ward, that these special people, thankfully, would care far too much for the welfare of their patients to ever consider walking away from them!

Having little else to do, I flicked open my iPad and 'Googled' the NHS and Lord Kerslake. I was astonished to read that His Lordship appeared in the Guardian Newspaper's list of the 'top one-hundred, most-influential people in the UK'. To me, however, he wasn't a household name. But I was interested in finding out why he believed his position was untenable?

Regarding the NHS, there were a myriad of websites, political comment and blogs. For a short time, I read one or two bits, though not enough to pretend expertise in the subject. I did, however, identify a recurring theme, in addition to the well documented financial issues.

It is endemic within the organisation that many staff are having to work extra shifts because there is a high level of absenteeism, due to what is suspected to be stress-related illnesses. If it is correct that this is a major cause of absenteeism, and that many wards apparently only function with 'Bank' staff, it does concern me that patient care, despite the best of intentions, is bound to suffer.

For what it's worth, I thought it right that Lord Kerslake should resign, provided he converts his principled action in to one of positivity. In my opinion, just making a statement and walking away does little, or anything, to better the situation that has been left behind. The Guardian list informed us that Lord Kerslake is a man of great influence. If that is so, then he should use his influence in securing the future sustainability of our precious NHS.

"I hope that makes sense to you, My Lord, because it does to me!"

The 'Today' programme, also interviewed a politician who rigorously supported the argument in favour of securing the UK's borders and drastically curtailing immigration once membership of the European Union was ended.

It was a matter of fact that I was being cared for by people from all over the world; France, Spain, Eastern Europe, India, the Philippines and Australia. People from all over the globe fulfil roles from consultancy through to ancillary in all facets of the Organisation. If the existing process of recruitment from abroad and the renewal of existing contracts of foreign staff were to be endangered, what would the implications be for patients of the NHS?

The elected representative for 'Little England', in my humble opinion, could do with a lesson in lateral thinking that might lead him to question his personal fantasy of an ideal world!

I croaked at the radio and waved my fist like a latter-day Tim Henman after scoring a point at Wimbledon. I was probably inaudible to others around me, but if not, it was likely that my rantings and actions would have been dismissed as fever or something.

"Listen to me, Rt. Hon. Twit M.P.! Am I standing at the bar, in my local, having a healthy debate among the alcohol fumes? No, as it happens, I am incarcerated in an NHS hospital bed, apparently unhealthy and desperately reliant on, and grateful to, my united nation of carers. Yes, I do have an axe to grind, and as these good people busy themselves around me, I have time to reflect on my situation. So, mate, as important as you think you are, don't rush your fences!"

Phew!! It was high time that I got off my proverbial soapbox and concentrated on getting myself better.

My headache seemed to have got a lot worse.

Hadn't the Doctor told me to avoid stressful situations? Perhaps It might have been more profitable to have listened to him rather than to Radio 4. I resolved, there and then, that I would refrain from starting each morning with a dose of the 'Today' programme.

Little did they know it, and if they had, it is likely that they would not have cared, but the listener statistics of Mr John Humphrys and his mates had just plummeted by one!

Chapter 4

The pain in the right-side of my head had become acute. This stroke was not going to let go of me as easily as I had expected. I just lay in bed holding my face and moaning.

"Surely to God someone can give me something to ease this pain," I whinged to anyone in the vicinity of my bed who would be prepared to listen, "after all, I am in a flipping hospital!"

The nurses and carers did listen, and were sympathetic, but they patiently explained to me that they were forbidden to prescribe any painkillers stronger than Paracetemol until after I had undergone an MRI scan.

An MRI scanner is a large tube that contains powerful magnets. The patient lies inside the tube during the scan. It can be used to examine almost any part of the body, including the spinal cord and brain. Even to me, though in the depth of despond, it was obvious and logical that my head and brain should be properly surveyed and analysed before further appropriate medication could be given. But rationality was not one of my strengths at this moment in time.

I had had a bad day and when Angela and some of the family visited that evening, I was not the best of company. They were obviously worried about me, but I must admit that one gets very selfish, when feeling ill, and all I was concerned about was the ruddy pain in my head. All attempts at conversation from my loved ones were greeted from me by moans and whinges. I was in pain and troubled by the bright lights and the inevitable noise on the Ward. Though I appreciated them visiting me, my only wish was for them to stop all the small talk and to do something about it! This was a seemingly impossible and irrational request, and their helplessness deserved better understanding. The little group around my bed was joined by one of the nursing assistants. Gina was an easy-going red head. She had a very warm and caring nature and always enjoyed a bit of banter. She was very kind, and supportive, to Angela too. She seemed always to be there for her when a comforting hug was urgently required. She stroked my head as she sympathetically discussed my situation with the family and reassured them that everything was under control before moving on to her next patient.

A short time afterwards, Gina reappeared.

"A side room has been vacated, but we've got to move fast!"

My bed immediately began to move as Gina, assisted by my grandson Asher, pushed it out of the bay, and within a couple of minutes I was the sole resident of 'Room Two'. It had been a difficult day, but now I felt settled and at peace, away from the turmoil of the ward. I don't think I have ever felt so grateful or more privileged. To my way of thinking, 'Room Two' was as sumptuous as a suite in the Savoy Hotel. Within a very short time, as Angela was displaying my growing collection of 'Get Well' cards around 'my' room, the door was opened and a porter attempted to push a bed, together with an incumbent patient, into my space. He stopped suddenly. "As if in an emergency", my driving test examiner would have said.

"Sorry, mate!" he said, addressing the assembled gathering as if they were a single being, "I've obviously got the wrong room." He pulled back and shut the door. It dawned on us that Gina had neither asked, nor sought, permission to remove me from the ward, and that my only chance of remaining in 'Room Two', undisturbed, would be to claim squatters' rights. Fortunately, this action was not deemed necessary as a short while later somebody had slotted a card, bearing the name Harold Lawrence, into the allotted space on the door. Gina had obviously stood her ground and fought my corner, bless her.

From the time the bed-push began from the Bay to Room Two, there hadn't been a single dull moment. But the night was still young and there was time for yet another twist in the tale.

"There can be only one Harold Lawrence, what are you doing here?" said a voice that I certainly recognised.

I turned towards the door and raised my head from the pillow to be greeted by the sight of a pyjama-clad figure bent over a Zimmer frame. It was Mal, a friend from my hometown, who I had known for quite thirty years.

"Blimey, Mal," I croaked, "what are you doing here?"

With hindsight, it was an exchange of words, rather than a conversation, totally void of imagination and originality. What the hell would we be doing here as patients in the Acute Stroke Unit? Perhaps we had both had a stroke?

Mal had gathered much more medical knowledge by far than me about his illness. All I knew about mine, at this moment in time, was that I had a bloody headache and my right eye was hurting, and as soon as they give me some painkillers that work, I'll be off home on Friday. However, Mal enlightened me that the Consultant had advised him that his stroke was relatively rare and was described as lateral medulla syndrome. Now, this rang a bell. They were the very words that the Consultant had used about me when discussing his suspicions with the students. He had also told me that it was a rare type of stroke, but there was one other patient in the ward that was being treated with the same symptoms.

"Flipping heck, Mal," I muttered, "it's you! We must have caught it off each other!"

Soon after, it was time for my visitors to leave. They each, in turn, bent over my prostrate frame and gave me a kiss. I waved farewell to them without opening my eyes.

It had been way beyond the bounds of a mundane hospital visit. I like many people have been party to one of those. It starts off all rather jolly.

"How are you? Your looks don't pity you!" (Ha! Ha! Ha!) "What's the food like? Is it better than the medicine?" (Ha! Ha! Ha!).

In my experience, each visitor speaks to the patient in turn

25

while the others sit around the patient's bed, for the next hour, exchanging small talk and surreptitiously glancing at their watches, trying not to yawn, and looking for an excuse to leave without appearing rude. Perhaps other cynics, like me, might recognise this description of a hospital visit.

But,

my visitors had had a hectic time, with hardly a minute in which to exchange small talk. I am certain that they must have felt it had been a long day. They must have been desperate for a cup of cocoa and an early night. As for me, I was just pleased to be left quietly, in my private suite, to nurse my headache. However, closing your eyes has no effect on the efficient running of the hospital machine.

"Sorry to disturb you but I 've got to take you down to Radiography."

With my eyes half-open, I looked up into the face of a hospital porter. Without any elaboration, he pushed me and the bed back through the open door that had welcomed us to 'Room Two', barely an hour previously. My head was throbbing, and I was in no mood to either question or protest, but I still managed to mutter, "Don't forget I've got squatters' rights" to the bemused man, who probably thought it was just befuddled ramblings typical of patients who have suffered a stroke.

I was whisked along silent hospital corridors, even the wheels of the bed were muffled by the rubber cladding on the floor. It had certainly been a bizarre evening. At visiting time, I had been surrounded by my worried loved-ones who, with the blessed connivance of Gina, had found me a room on my own, then I had met up with Mal, now I am being conveyed through a silent world by a silent porter to God knows where. Hospital is not the place for a control-freak, unless he is trying to kick the habit. It is the institution that controls and directs. I was embarked on this journey having, I am sure, been the subject of an exclusive discussion elsewhere and to suit the agenda of others. That was not a complaint, only an observation.

In a short while, we finally reached our destination, and I was pushed into a brightly lit room and was greeted, in foreign accents, by two white coated technicians. My erstwhile companion and bed-pusher retreated from the room without any comment, and as he left, I heard his pager beep, which was probably advising him of his next errand.

The radiologists manoeuvred me off the bed and on to the table of the MRI scanner. They were very efficient, but it did occur to me that they were certainly not smiley folk. I decided that this might be a cultural thing but then reasoned that they were probably nearing the end of a twelve-hour shift and by now a warm bedside manner would be quite low on their priority list.

"Put on these earphones, please. Here is an escape button for you to hold. Press it if you have a need to come out of the scanner. We will stop the scan immediately and take you out. Please hold your arms to your side. We will now slide you into the tube and commence your scan"

Up to this point I had been holding my head in a futile attempt to stop the aching. Now this was no longer possible, and I began to panic as it appeared to become more intense. With hindsight, I am sure that this was psychological, but it was certainly a nervy time. I had only been in the machine a minute and my right thumb was already poised and twitching over the escape button. But there really was no point. I'd only be delaying things, and both I and the medics knew that this scan was essential. Suddenly the noise of a road drill shattered the silence and vibrated above my head! Having had no prior briefing, combined with the pain in my head, I admit that I was rather shaken! However, I gritted my teeth and guessed that it would soon be over. After what seemed like a very long five minutes, the 'drilling' ceased, and all was silent.

Thank goodness for that, I thought, just as well I didn't push the button, I'll be out of here in a sec. But I continued to lay there. What are they waiting for? Ignorance may be bliss, but it can also be a curse. The drilling began again. I learned quickly that there was a pattern, five minutes drilling, five minutes rest and this continued, in total, for forty-five minutes! I just about coped, but I am sure that I would have coped better if I had been informed more about the procedure.

"Nobody told me that you worked for the SAS" I said, forcing a smile.

"Pardon?" replied the technician, "We work for NHS."

"Are you sure?" I continued, "I thought this was the point that the SAS took over to find out how much torture patients are able to absorb"

Without betraying a semblance of comprehension, he shrugged his shoulders, and with a note of finality in his voice, he responded,

"No, NHS!"

My attempt at English humour had truly fallen on stony ground. I estimated that he was approximately the same age as my daughters, so I really should not have been surprised by his reactions to my perceived witticisms.

Before long, it was with a sense of relief, that I was returned to the peace and solitude of 'Room Two'. The Night Sister administered a dose of an extra strong painkiller, together with three or four cardboard urine bottles, and tucked me in for the night.

I probably had my best night's sleep since being admitted. No pain, no noise, and in splendid isolation. I slept like a baby. Interrupted only by the 'Obs Patrol' every four hours... oh, and a couple of pees!

Chapter 5

It was the clanking of the housekeepers' trolleys, as they went about their task of serving breakfast, that brought me back in to full consciousness and to the realisation that isolation may not always be splendid. Patients are asked to select from the breakfast menu before dawn, although daylight and darkness make little impression on the routine workings of a hospital ward. There were the inevitable raised voices as the first meal of the day was distributed to a ward of people, many of whom, due to their strokes, have difficulty in comprehending or communicating.

Mimi, a cheerful, little, bespectacled, Spanish lady, poked her head round my door.

"'Ello, what you doing 'ere? You not had breakfast? You been missed, no worry, what you like? I'll get!"

"I moved here last night. I'd like porridge, toast and marmalade please. Thanks luv!"

She disappeared, returning soon afterwards with food for a fortunate squatter.

I was back in the routine, and before long health care assistant, Erica, came in to introduce herself and told me that she would be looking after me, and would I like to have a shower.

Wow, a shower!

Earlier, I had also had a quick visit from one of the physiotherapist team who advised me that I had been programmed, mid-morning, to spend an hour in the gymnasium.

A shower followed by a visit to the Gym. Was I, at long last, back on track to normality?

I was not feeling as dizzy as I had been, so I was sure that, with Erica's assistance and the support of a walking frame, I would be able to successfully negotiate my way to the bathroom.

I dug out my wash bag and towels from the bedside locker,
then swung my legs off the bed and for the first time, since my
earlier aborted attempt, my feet touched the floor. From a sitting
position, I pushed myself in to a standing position.

"No problem", I thought, then, "who-oh!"

Erica grabbed my arm, steadied me and placed my hands on the
walking frame. I attempted a couple of steps but felt extremely
wobbly and came over nauseous. I panicked as I struggled to
control both sensations.

From seemingly nowhere, Erica produced a wheelchair, and made
an executive decision that it would provide a far safer conveyance
for this bathroom trip. She sensibly ignored my protestation that
I would be perfectly OK as soon as I had retrieved my 'land-legs'
and was not at all impressed by my promise that I would not fall
over and squash her. She pushed me along the corridor to the
shower room, where I was undressed and gently manoeuvred
from the wheelchair to a plastic chair placed strategically next to
the 'hand- held' shower. She tested the temperature of the water
against my arm.

"A bit hotter, please", I said. She increased the temperature, "it's
still too cold" I said.

"It's as hot as it will go" Erica replied. At that moment some water
splashed on to the other side of my body.

"Gawd! That's hot!!!" I exclaimed. Realisation dawned on me that I
had apparently lost the sensation of hot and cold down the left-
hand side of my body. I decided that I would have to manage this
situation very carefully in future if I was to avoid ending up in a
burns-unit. Kindly, Erica reassured me and said that all would get
better in time.

The now defunct News of the World used to display a strapline boasting that within their pages "All human life is there". That may or not have been true, but there is no doubting the veracity of this statement when applied to the NHS. Its ethos and success depend wholly on the fact that people matter, and from my own experience there exists no other institution where this theory is so clearly and successfully put into practice. I cannot for the life of me think of any other organisation where people from so many nationalities and backgrounds are placed in a situation where they care for and rely on each other to such a degree. It is truly a melting pot. Religious, political and racial boundaries do not exist. It seems rather perverse to me that it is in hospital, a place where in the ideal world nobody would want to be, one learns and appreciates how an ideal world should be.

There is no point in denying, however, as it is a fact, that whatever our culture, we are all but flesh and blood, and as part of the hospital community, whether patient or carer, we are certainly reminded from day to day that we all have our fair share of frailties and vulnerabilities. Certainly, there are highs and lows, laughter and tears, but there is also the shared delight and rejoicing in one another's progress and little victories, integrated with empathy and sympathy, for those struggling to overcome challenges. We are all human, patients and carers, and even those with the most gregarious of personalities are prone to moods. Sometimes we may feel 'on top of the world' and at other times we are 'down in the dumps' and feeling a bit grumpy. It is too easy to be judgemental on such occasions. It was my privilege, as a stroke patient, to find for myself another definition of the N.H.S.

Nurses (without) Halos are still Saints!

(I implied a modicum of poetic licence as, by definition, nurses, included all the carers, be they porter or physician.)

Erica was such a lovely, kind person, hard-working and caring, as too are many of her colleagues, and she always goes that extra yard for her patients. During the twenty minutes or so spent completing my ablutions, I took the opportunity to get to know the person behind the caring professional. She is a Filipino, married to an Englishman and the mother of a young daughter. The little girl is looked after, when not in childcare, by each parent whilst the other is working. Erica's husband is also a care worker, and she inferred that the family budget was quite tight. She has a bright personality and enjoyed a joke, though she readily admitted having had, at times, difficulty understanding the English sense of humour when she first came to live and work in the country. She had obviously learned fast! She told me that her mother and father squeezed a meagre living from working a small farm. She has one sister and two brothers, and growing up in the provinces of the Philippines, though unsophisticated, was a happy time. She left home, as a teenager, to work as a nurse in Singapore, where she stayed for three years before moving to London. She said that moving away from home at such a young age had been traumatic and that she had been very frightened. Her sister also left and went abroad in order to nurse. As is customary within their culture, they both sent home some of their wages to help support their family. She told me, excitedly, that she was planning a visit to introduce her parents to their granddaughter for the first time since she was born. She had accepted, regrettably, that there was little prospect of ever returning home to the Philippines to live but was grateful that her little girl had bright prospects growing up in the UK. Despite her happy disposition, I detected a momentary sadness in her eyes as she spoke of her family and admitted there were many occasions when she felt very homesick.

I wished, at that moment, that the xenophobic MP who I had listened to being interviewed on the BBC, together with those that shared his philosophy, could have been party to our conversation and had, like me, the privilege to listen to Erica's story. Rather than threaten to exile the likes of her, it might dawn on them how essential their work is within the NHS and decide that a vote of thanks might be more appropriate. But then it was more likely that Erica's Mum and Dad's pigs might fly first!

Showered, shaved and feeling a 'new man', even if a bit of a wobbly one, I was pushed back to my bed. It was only a matter of five minutes before my presence was required by the physiotherapists. Two athletic young ladies hauled me to my feet and assessed that though I would be taken to the gym by wheelchair, I should attempt to walk back with the aid of a walking frame.

I was pushed into a room that contained a table, an exercise bike and a set of parallel bars. There were also three other patients, two men and a woman, to whom I was formally introduced by name. This, to me, seemed an unnecessary protocol because, apart from nodding and smiling, my patient colleagues were unable to converse with one another and none seemed to be anywhere near as keen as I was to be there. We were sat around the table together and were set exercises that involved, first, rolling balls to each other, then throwing them. As my initial throw whistled past the ear of the gentlemen opposite me, I realised that there was little wrong with my strength, but that my co-ordination still required work in progress! One of the physiotherapists' suggested that I spend fifteen minutes on the bike. I suspected that this decision was made in the interests of health and safety. Not mine, I might add, but certainly that of my fellow patients. If my throw had been half an inch to the left, it might have set the poor man's recovery back six months.

I worked hard. After the allotted time, the read-out on the little monitor, attached to the handlebars, declared that I had ridden four point five kilometres and I had put in ninety-seven per cent effort. I was sure it was wrong, as to me it felt more like ten kilometres and at least one hundred and fifty per cent effort.

Next, I was pushed in the wheelchair to the parallel bars and asked to stand up between them at one end, walk four paces to the other end then walk backwards to the start point.

Piece of cake, I thought, but was it? Like heck! After just one step I found myself clinging on to the bars so tightly that it was a miracle that they didn't splinter. The room started to spin around, and I abruptly sat back to the safety of the chair.

"Oh dear, will I ever be able to walk again?" I bleated.

"Yes, you will, you still have strength in all your limbs, it is just a question of training your brain to restore your balance. We will give you a list of exercises that you will be able to do whilst laying on your bed, as well as further time spent in the gym" said the physio, cheerfully.

"No problem, then," said I.

Despite my exertions, I was determined to keep to the original plan and walk back to the ward on my walking frame. I was not going to allow my negative experience on the bars to weaken my resolve. With a physiotherapist on each side of me, and one behind, pushing the empty wheelchair, I slowly walked, with the aid of the walking frame, across the room, out of the door and into the corridor. It seemed a very long way back to my room, and it felt like I was running a marathon whilst constantly being motivated and kept focussed by the vocal encouragement and support from my team of helpers. I virtually collapsed on to my bed. I was totally fatigued yet, in that moment, I basked in a surge of heightened satisfaction. It was going to be a long haul, but the extreme pain in my head had disappeared, thank God, and the numbness down the right side of my face had receded slightly. It certainly felt like progress.

By now I had been a resident of The Acute-Stroke Ward for nine days, and it occurred to me that this was five days longer than Doctor Egg had suggested. I mentioned this fact to the ward Sister. Obviously, she did not know the stroke specialist by the alias that I had bestowed upon him, but agreed, that with the use of a little imagination, it would be possible to describe him as 'egg-shaped'. I had hoped that she would be able to teach me how to pronounce his name correctly, but disappointedly she said that she, too, had difficulty in getting her tongue round it! Whatever the good doctor's name, she was adamant that, 'patient discharge' was never the sole decision of one individual. The whole stroke team had to agree, which included the physiotherapists and the other therapists.

To be honest, I knew that I was in no way ready to go home, and was comforted and reassured to be told that my fate did not rest on the word of one person, but on the consensus of a committee

Mind you, if it works to the same rules that apply to a jury, did that mean I could be stuck in hospital for months whilst waiting for a majority verdict?

I had had an active day, and by the time Angela arrived at visiting time, I was as fatigued as I probably would have been had I just ended a twelve-hour shift mining a seam of coal. However, Angela looked stressed and even more tired, poor thing. She had been besieged by telephone calls, had the additional onus of having to keep on top of the day to day problems at home, plus a thirty-mile round trip twice a day for the past nine days.

Sitting in my hospital bed being fed, watered and generally cared for, it seemed to me that I certainly had the better part of the deal.

I had other visitors during the afternoon session and Angela was joined by members of the family in the evening. I was delighted to see them all, and my tiredness seemed to evaporate as I guess I played to the gallery, in my efforts to be hospitable, as well as, dare I say it, as entertaining as it is possible to be whilst under the auspices of the NHS. Despite warnings, received from my carers, that as a stroke patient, I should avoid undue excitement and situations that might cause fatigue, which is an inherent feature of a stroke, I readily admit to encouraging my visitors to linger longer than perhaps was medically appropriate.

As the evening wore on it was noticeable that my voice was becoming very husky, and I noticed that my capacity to swallow seemed to be eroding. It seemed painful and difficult on the left side of my throat. More importantly, the dreaded headache was returning as if to avenge my stupidity in believing that I was impervious to my physical frailties. I was sure that a good night's sleep is all that the doctor would order, and for the second time within a week, I gestured farewell to Angela and the family with my head buried in the pillows and my eyes tight shut.

Chapter 6

One of the most important events in the daily hospital routine is 'Handover'. This is the time of the day when one shift ends, and another takes over. The conditions and problems, if any, of individual patients are exchanged and discussed with a certain amount of urgency. It is fair to say that, after a long and highly active shift, tired carers are anxious to sign off and get back home. But no one can leave before all the formalities are completed. You might suggest that I should get a life, but I admit that I found 'Handover' great fun!

Day-staff meet night-staff, in the morning, and information is disseminated amid the general melee and confusion. Tucked up in my little room, I listened to exuberant greetings, updates on the weather and traffic problems. It is a little window on the outside world that is opened twice a day; morning and evening.

I was born during the War, and at that time, the Ministry of Information (I think it was) were concerned about enemy spies operating in the country. They used to design and issue posters to warn the public. One of them had the slogan 'Walls have Ears'. They could have done with one of these pinned to the Ward noticeboard, as the warning is as pertinent today as it was, way back in those dark hours of conflict.

The staff decided to conduct their handover meeting in the corridor, directly outside my room.

The door was slightly ajar, and I found myself tuned in to the distinctive voice of a member of staff that I had recognised from my first morning in hospital. This person appeared to be playing a star role in the handover forum, making far more impact than she seemed to do whilst on duty. As I listened, I decided that she would have made a good candidate on Alan Sugar's television show 'The Apprentice'. I imagined that she would give a good account of herself when under scrutiny in the boardroom, but for the life of me, I found it difficult to understand how she managed to accumulate her knowledge.

As I listened, I realised that she was waxing lyrical about a patient whom I knew intimately. Yes, it appeared that she was conducting an analytical discourse on patient Harold Lawrence, or 'Room Two', as she professionally identified him!

I was nonplussed as I was aware that her 'in depth' profile was based on one brief meeting on the morning of my admission which I remembered clearly.

She had asked me whether I was able to wash myself. I was determined not to appear an invalid. Of course, I was still in a state of shock and still coming to terms with my newly acquired status of stroke patient along with my sudden, and totally unexpected, loss of dignity. In fairness, it was only a short time ago that I had assumed myself to be, both mentally and physically, fit. It was far from my thinking that I would soon be in my present predicament. I suppose it had all happened so quickly that I was still in denial.

I boldly, though unwisely, asserted that I was quite capable of performing my own ablutions. She presented me with a bowl of warm water with some immersed wipes and a towel before pulling together the curtains around the bed. I presumed to protect me from the prying eyes of strangers. I was left alone. My pride was intact, and I had commenced a ham-fisted attempt at washing myself. In fact, more water penetrated the bed sheets than came close to moisturising my face.

It was almost another hour later before she returned. She was jolly enough as she whisked away the bowl of, now cold, water, and the unused towel. She had retreated through a gap in the curtains, without a backward glance. As she left the slightly smelly, but wiser, patient, she gave neither a hint, nor any clue, that she was in any way aware that he was wallowing, like a hippopotamus, in his swampy bed.

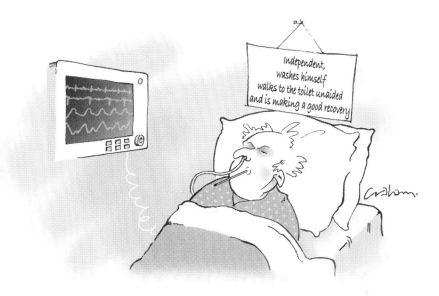

Independent, washes himself walks to the toilet unaided and is making a good recovery

You can probably imagine my astonishment when I overheard her submission to the meeting. According to her 'input' to Handover, "Room Two is independent, washes himself, walks to the toilet unaided, and is making a good recovery."

It sounded as if I was being dismissed as self-sufficient. I would not have been at all surprised if she had concluded her statement with the words "... for a malingerer."

The fact was that I had now been in hospital ten days, some good some bad, and as I was still at a point of my recovery where I had occasional headaches, stumbled to the toilet with the aid of a walking frame and the supervision of a care assistant, and my co-ordination and balance still being worked on by the physiotherapists. I think it was fair to say that I had known a greater level of independence than she assumed I was enjoying at present.

I lay in my room quietly worrying that I would be sent home. You would think that I would be overjoyed by the prospect, but I knew that I was far from being my old self.

Later that morning, I confessed to the Ward Sister that I had been listening in to the handover meeting and voiced my concerns that I had overheard what had been said about me. At my request, she produced my file. She read it carefully and after a couple of minutes, she looked up and smiled at me.

"You have no need to worry, Harold. Everything is under control. Nobody has been influenced by anybody."

Chapter 7

According to the entry in my diary, on Friday the 15th December, I had planned that I would be shaking a tin for charities outside Tesco to be followed by, that evening, the Rotary Club's Christmas party.

With hindsight, it would have been more appropriate if it had been amended to a 'one-liner';

"All aboard the white-knuckle ride! Fasten your safety belt!" The day had started as was usual. Breakfast was served. I ate a bowl of porridge and drank a small carton of orange juice. But then, I found, to my surprise, and despite prolonged chewing, I was unable to swallow a bite of toast and marmalade. I tried to wash it down with a sip of water, but this only added to the problem and I started to choke. With tears running down my face, I felt a surge of panic. I spat the contents of my mouth into a bowl. I then took another sip of water only to find that I was unable to swallow this too and it also had to be spat out. To my horror, realisation dawned that I had completely lost my ability to swallow, even to the extent that my saliva was also building up in my mouth and had to be similarly dispatched. I pushed the emergency button and a nurse provided me with several cardboard bowls to spit into. She told me that my swallow would be monitored throughout the day. This new development in my condition was very frightening. Apparently, this is a not uncommon symptom, but I was advised that it is unusual to lose the ability to swallow so long after the initial event.

I had to programme my mind to cope with this unexpected direction that my illness had taken. I was mentally entering a chapter of my life that was way beyond anything I had previously experienced.

The most positive thing I could do to lighten the moment was to seek out the humour in the situation. For some reason, my mind flashed back many years to when I stayed at the home of Evan, a friend of my father's, who lived in the mining village of Nantymoel, which is situated in the South Wales valley of Ogmore.

He was, himself, an ex-miner and had had to retire from the pit since he suffered from the lung condition, pneumoconiosis, which is caused by the inhalation of coal-dust, and commonly suffered by miners. To ease his problem, it necessitated in him, from time to time, coughing up mucus from his lungs. He had developed a disconcerting habit of spitting into the burning coal fire, but luckily, for those within spitting distance, his delivery was always accurately placed from wherever he was sitting in the room. I seem to remember that nobody took exception to, nor even noticed, this unhygienic habit. It was a story that I could have dined out on, but didn't, as it was probably an inappropriate anecdote to introduce at the table!

Anyway, I wrote 'spittoon', boldly, with a black felt-tip pen, on the side of the cardboard receptacles that I had been given for the purpose and I resolved, there and then, to emulate Evan and become an expert and accurate practitioner.

Despite this recent development, the medics had previously arranged an agenda of events to keep me amused, and they were not going to be deflected from their course by a little swallowing problem. I was becoming convinced that stroke treatment is like being at war. There are hours of ennui punctuated with momentary rushes of high adrenaline tinged, on occasions, with a little bit of fear. Stroke care, I think, cannot possibly be a precise science.

Having just been advised by a health assistant that I was due for a shower, a portly member of the Occupational Therapy team turned up and announced that he wanted to observe me washing myself. A bowl of water was produced for my use, and my audience of one settled himself comfortably in a chair and opened his notebook. I half expected him to peer at me through a pair of gilded opera glasses. I managed to perform all the acts of my ablutions to his satisfaction although, amid all this impromptu theatre, I missed out on a shave.

As the day progressed, I noticed that the medical staff began to emphasise and sympathise with me over my lack of a swallow. Two doctors appeared at the door and asked me how long I had been unable to swallow and another couple of questions about my general health. They nodded their heads wisely at my responses and suggested that they would like the 'Speech and Language' department to have a look at me... "But as it is now Friday – you probably won't be seen before Monday..." (Help!!!)

In the meantime, I decided that I would continue to practice and improve my skills at the spittoon. However, as I have already alluded, there's never a dull moment in hospital, provided you are prepared to wait for an hour or two.

Staff nurse Sadie introduced herself and requested my permission to do some blood tests. The consequences should I have declined did not enter my head, but after clearing the saliva from my mouth in to the spittoon, I replied, "Why not? You're beautiful and I might still have some blood left, so I can't immediately think of a better person to give it to." I knew that my smooth tongue would get me into trouble one day and today was that day. After three failed attempts Staff Nurse Sadie advised me that she had only qualified a month previously, and that taking blood was not one of her better skills. She apologised and said she would get one of her colleagues who, apparently, had had many more years of practice! An hour later, Sadie reappeared and advised me that she needed to insert a cannula into a vein in my arm so that drugs could be pumped into my system, now that I was unable to swallow. This time she was successful on her third attempt. I decided that Sadie, like a darts player, sometimes needed 'a sighter' before hitting the target, though prior to this she had had no problem pushing a suppository filled with Aspirin up my back passage, without a rehearsal! She made no more mention of the blood tests, and I was not about to remind her.

It was, so far, turning out to be one of the strangest days in my post-stroke life. It had not been short of surprises, but its store was far from exhausted and Sadie, clearly, was not yet finished with me.

"Harold, I have got to fit an NGT, have you had this procedure before?" she asked.

"I don't think so Sadie, what is an NGT? You have to remember that I'm newer to this malarkey than even you are." I replied.

"It's a Nasal Gastric Tube. As you are unable to swallow, it is inserted, via your nose, into your stomach so that you are able to receive nutrition." She started to immediately push a plastic tube into my nostril, accompanied by the instruction, "swallow!" Perhaps she had forgotten that this was impossible and the very reason I was having this damned procedure in the first place. After some jiggling, retching and a dash of panic, the NGT was finally in place. I was then told that I had to have a trip to the radiology department for an X-ray to make sure that the device had been fitted correctly.

What with the failure in taking blood, and three attempts before the cannula was successfully inserted, perhaps it is fair to say, that I could only describe my optimism that the NGT had landed in the right place, as cautious? However, the suppository had certainly hit the mark, so when I said "Thank God" after the Radiographer gave a positive response, perhaps I was being a tad unfair to Nurse Sadie.

Back on the ward I was attached to a large packet of 'Nutrisa'. One of the care assistants very kindly sympathised with me, but I replied "Breakfast, lunch and dinner all out of a bag. No more time wasted having to pick up knives, forks, spoons and cups. No more time wasted chewing. More time for conversation – surely, this is the life!"

I tried to keep negativity out of my mind. Though, I admit that it did occur to me that if I was still wired up to meals-in-a-bag by Easter, a visit from Doctor Egg might be the closest I would get to having a festive treat.

Chapter 8

Over the years you meet all types of people and personalities.
When I first left school, I started work in a bank. One of my
new colleagues, though little older than myself, seemed super-
confident and I used to be somewhat inhibited by him. I don't
think he meant it. He was self-assured, but rarely smiled, could be
abrupt, and was undoubtedly efficient. He was all a bit too much
for a latter-day schoolboy like me, who was still more comfortable
playing football with his mates than in the adult world of work. He
was not a person that was easy to warm to. He rarely allowed a
glimpse of his life away from the office, although strangely, to my
mind, he could be quite inquisitive about yours. I tried hard to get
to know him better, but inevitably failed. Yet, others used to say
that he was friendlier towards me than to anyone!

Where is all this leading?

Well, in the acute stroke ward, fifty-eight years later, I met
up with a similar person. He was busy, efficient, a bit lacking
in 'bedside-manner', and certainly intense. He was the Ward
Sister. Furthermore, he spoke with an accent that betrayed his
French nationality. I have an annoying habit, as far as my wife is
concerned, of always giving people nick-names. My first thought
was to name him Sister Intense. But then I thought back to my
employment in the Bank. I recalled that all the senior staff had to
be referred to as 'Sir.' I thought Sister Intense might enjoy being
called Sir Intense But, my imagination was now gathering the
momentum of a run-away train. Hadn't I scraped a pass in GCE
French, and now considered myself a bit of a linguist? Of course,
the French word for sister was soeur and that was pronounced the
same as 'Sir'. Perfect! I thought, Soeur Intense he shall be!"

Having earlier bade farewell to my visitors and family that included
all my grandsons, who I will not list by name in case it gives the
impression that I don't love them all equally! I was in a good
mood, as I generally was, after visiting time. In all institutions,
whether it is the District General, Rest-a-While Care Home or
Wormwood Scrubs, visiting times are awaited by the inmates with

great expectation and pleasure. Boundaries seem to miraculously expand, as fresh faces and voices bring news and gossip from beyond the walls. However, it will still take a lot to convince me that visiting the sick isn't an alien task from the perspective of the poor visitors!

Though somewhat isolated, I was becoming comfortable and contented in my 'private' room, and I settled down to watch a bit of television before 'lights-out'. I have always tried to avoid becoming complacent, in my life, because it is so easy to be jolted from it. This time was to prove no exception.

Soeur Intense whirled into my room.

Without any preamble, he said, "I will be moving you from this room to 'Bed One' in E-bay." He looked around the room at my growing collection of 'Get Well' cards, and gesturing dismissively with a wave of his arm, continued, "there will be no space for these. We will collect them all up and your wife can take them back home with her."

It was a fait accompli, and he broached no argument. "OK." I responded lamely as, in an instant, my bed was pushed out of my squat and along the corridor to E-bay.

The minute hand on the clock seemed to confuse itself with that of the hour hand. My first night in E-bay stretched elastically before me and was intermittently punctuated by the groans, moans and shouts from my suffering ward-mates. I managed to doze-off, in between the inevitable interruptions of the Obs Patrol.

It felt as if my elite suite had been replaced by a dormitory in the NHS's version of a 'Boot Camp, in order to toughen me up for the next stage of my recovery.

At an unseemly hour, 'Carer Cara' had stood at the entrance and introduced herself, as the carer to the six elderly gentlemen in E-bay. I supposed that this was challenge enough, without the added complication of them all being stroke patients. I had already, having been forced to listen to them throughout the night, and as is my way, renamed my fellow patients Grumpy Mal, Allawry John, Mister Sleepy, Sir Surgical Sock, Effllyn Gethin, and in the interest of fairness, named myself Wonky Wotsit. I believed that it would be a difficult shift ahead for 'Carer Cara' and her colleagues. I subsequently discovered, from Cara, that she was an extreme sports enthusiast which made me surmise that practising her profession was probably just another event. But surely competing in a triathlon or a marathon in the Sahara Desert must be a damn sight easier?

I was brought to full consciousness by the raised voice of my old friend Mal, tucked up in the bed opposite, who was grumpily blaming 'Carer Cara' for waking him up.

"You don't need to be like that, I'm only here to help you!" Cara said, under her breath, as she moved on to the next patient. She was obviously not too happy about starting her day on the wrong foot, and as I was sure that it was important that harmonious relationships should be restored as a matter of urgency, I called out to her.

"Don't let grumpy old Mal upset you, Cara, he's a very nice man when you get to know him and always cheers up by the middle of the morning. By the way, my name's Harold, better known as 'Wonky Wotsit' and I'm very pleased that you are looking after us." She laughed, Mal laughed, and team spirit seemed to have been restored.

What I had not anticipated, at this moment, was that I was to be Cara's first major problem of the day.

I desperately wanted to go to the toilet, but as I was not allowed to visit the bathroom without assistance, and 'Carer Cara' was preoccupied with one of the other patients, I did not wish to pester her. It was not a major emergency. I had a supply of urine bottles and was quite happy to use one. What I had forgotten was that I had had the foot of my mattress raised slightly during the night whilst I was struggling to find a comfortable position in my effort to counteract insomnia. I gratefully relieved myself. Then I experienced a warm sensation. To my horror and embarrassment, realisation dawned that I was sitting in a puddle of wee that had flowed back out of the bottle. When in hospital, loss of dignity is par for the course and any inhibitions are soon disregarded, but this was a situation that I had brought upon myself, aided only by my ignorance of bedding technology. Despite my earlier reticence, I called for Cara's assistance. Though I tried to make light of the matter I felt humiliated and ashamed. But Cara was a 'Carer-Extraordinaire', and she dealt with the situation, calmly, expertly, humorously and kindly. To say that I was appreciative would have been a woeful understatement.

Bedding quickly changed and dressing gown donned to cover my modesty, she decided that a refreshing shower should be the first order of the day. With Cara's assistance I managed to 'Zimmer' myself to the bathroom but, as I entered, the room suddenly whirly gigged! I flattened the palms of my hands against the wall, in order to steady myself, as Cara, a little bit panicked, held on to me. Luckily the stroke had not taken any strength from my arms or legs and I was able to avoid falling over.

It really had not been an auspicious start to the day. Perhaps it was proof that I needed more rest than I had been afforded on my first night in E bay. In my present frame of mind, I would have been delighted to have sold my bed in E-bay, on eBay to the first bidder!

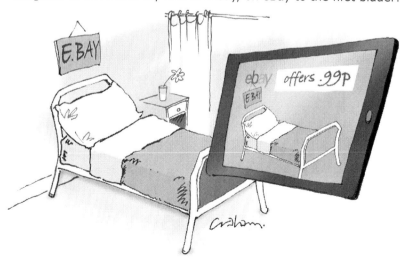

I soon recovered from my giddy-turn and a jolly interesting shower followed. 'Carer Cara' and I discussed road traffic accidents (RTA's), motor Insurance claims, holidays and travel insurance. Our conversation widened even further to subjects that varied from 'running in the Himalayas', 'the Marathon de Sable', to trekking along the 'South West Coastal Path' and the 'Wainwright Coast to Coast Walk'. All the while I was soaped, scrubbed, dried and shaved.

As I slowly and deliberately made my way back to my bed, I felt rejuvenated and fully prepared to face whatever was to be the next adventure that the NHS had up its sleeve for me.

It was Sunday, and unless an emergency occurred, routine procedures were not programmed so the morning period was effectively the quiet before the storm of extended visiting hours due to commence at 2 pm.

For me, it was an opportunity to write up a few notes and thereby reflect upon my situation. It is probably a bit cavalier to suggest that having a stroke is interesting, but I admit that this was the first time in my life that I had considered, for example, how the human brain is wired. I supposed, normally, that if you spent your waking hours obsessed with such a subject, you would be considered by your fellow man as 'a bit of a nut-case'. But here I was, sitting in a hospital ward feeling quite fortunate. I still had all my mental faculties intact. The numbness on the right side of my face and the inability to distinguish between hot and cold down the left of my body, reliance on the nasal gastric tube for nutrition and my struggle to balance and co-ordinate would all be OK, in good time, once my brain had successfully rewired itself!

One other thing, I had lost a certain amount of power in my voice which had also acquired a resonance that to me sounded croaky but one of the nurses described as "very sexy".

"Yes," I replied, "I am planning a new career in Hollywood."

Chapter 9

Since my admission to hospital, I had become even more ego-centric than usual. I suppose it was due, in part, to my cultivated, strong survival instinct. Had I been aboard the good ship Birkenhead, when it floundered, I suspect that the historic command would have been "Harold and Children first!"

Though I had been disappointed to exchange the relative peace and quiet of my exclusive 'Room Two' for the hustle, bustle and noise of E-bay. My first disturbed and sleep-deprived night was certainly a wake-up call! I was now sharing space with five other stroke survivors, all male and, as I surmised, in their seventies or older. Whoever we were, wherever we'd come from, whether rich or poor, one soon learned that 'Stroke' is the great leveller. It is predatory, stealthily stalking its prey before striking without mercy, leaving its victim frightened, confused, impaired and facing an uncertain future. All of us patients were having to come to terms with the situation and were struggling with various challenges. Of course, it was easy for me to respect, identify and be grateful for the special role that the professional carers played in the process of my recovery, but what was not so obvious was the important part my fellow patients also played.

Communication between patients, in a conversational sense, is limited, if not impossible, in a stroke unit. However, by observing and listening, I soon learned about the personalities and characters of those around me. I found it remarkable how, instinctively, I empathised and identified with erstwhile strangers to whom formal introductions seemed superfluous. The word 'love' is possibly a noun too far, but there is no doubt that I developed an affection for the inmates of E Bay, way beyond my wildest expectations. Yes, they were unwell and only shadows of their healthy selves, and at times they could be disruptive and annoying, but they all shared, during the long days and nights, snapshots of their true selves and humour. They may not have realised it, but they were certainly major players in making my extended stay in hospital much easier to tolerate.

Allawry John's philosophies, opinions and actions, were widely scattered around the ward, but only rarely directed at individuals. The stroke had left him with an irrationality that bordered upon a persecution complex. He was convinced, in his confusion, that the NHS was conspiring with a family friend to rob him of all his money and organise activities designed "to bump me orf!" He complained a lot, but in such a way that he entertained, rather than caused offence. Most of his interactions were with the nurses when he wasn't articulating loudly to himself.

"You certainly do love your bunnies, John" said the staff nurse, by way of conversation as she walked past his bed, which together with his bedside locker was cluttered with cuddly toys and a plastic night light that were all rabbit shaped.

"I love wild rabbits," Allawry John said, "they are furry and cuddly. I've got no time for them tame ones, though, because they are inclined to get eaten by weasels!" he said emphatically.

He seamlessly changed the subject.

"Are they going to turn off my life support?"

"As you are not on life support, I think that is highly unlikely Darling!"

"But I've read that they do it at Rampton. When am I going to have my pills?"

"You've had them, I watched you take them."

"I think you are lying; this hospital is conspiring to rob me of all my money then kill me orf!"

The staff nurse calmly reassured him that nothing of the sort was going to happen to him, and his agitation quickly subsided.

"You are like one of them nurses that I see walking up the hill from the bus. You're a saucy seal!"

The nurse giggled as she continued with her tasks. But A-J was still not finished.

"I blame the Conservatives." he said. "They've messed everything up!"

This last remark acted like a cattle prod into the ribs of the dozing 'Grumpy Mal'. He opened his eyes wide and shouted, "Typical! Always blame the poor old Conservatives...if ever Corbyn gets in to power you'll know what a mess is!"

"Blimey", I thought, "a political argument in a Stroke ward? I don't believe it." I mustered up as much volume as was possible with my newly acquired husky voice and called out to the nurse. "Do you agree Nurse that it is entirely inappropriate to argue politics in the stroke unit? Flipping heck, it'll be religion next!"

She giggled again, agreed with me and pretended to tell them off. It was all good fun.

I have already mentioned my habit of dolling out nick names. Besides A-J and Grumpy Mal, I was blessed, and had the pleasure to share with two other great characters, Effllyn Gethin and Sir Surgical Sock. Both were colourful and quite capable of adding a little disruption of their own when the mood took them.

One of the effects of stroke can be aphasia. This is a condition that causes the patient to have difficulty using language, and the ability to speak. It also affects understanding.

Being a native of Wales, I am sure Effllyn Gethin, in happier circumstances would, like most of his countrymen, be eloquent in his use of language. Therefore, I could easily understand his frustrations when he was trying to communicate with the nurses. Despite his efforts to articulate, he only managed to emit unintelligible noises. He would continuously call out to the staff in varying degrees of urgency and volume, "Grr mea er be de yer..."

"No, sweetheart, don't worry, you are not going to wet the bed, you're fitted with a catheter," was a typical response repeated many times over the course of a day.

But I shall always remember him fondly and be forever grateful to him for providing me with a true belly laugh. It was after lights out, and I was struggling to get comfortable and settle down to sleep, neither of which ever came easily for me. Effllyn Gethin, because he had had a fall and was quite badly bruised, had to be turned over in bed at regular intervals. This manoeuvre was usually completed without causing the patient any trauma, but sometimes, depending on the team of carers, the process would not always go quite so smoothly, and then the poor bloke would obviously be in a certain amount of pain.

From behind the privacy curtains drawn around his bed, 'turning' was in progress.

"Grr mea er be de yer," complained Effllyn Gethin. "grr mea er be de yer!" he complained more loudly, then totally frustrated, he shouted in a voice as richly resonant as a Welsh tenor, "Why doesn't someone fuckin' listen to me!!!...grr mea er be de yer..."

I couldn't restrain my laughter.

"Are you OK, Harold?" said a member of the 'turning team' on hearing my apparent gurgling outside the curtained bed space.

"No problem, just suffering from a surfeit of humour. Should be fine once my ribs stop aching," I croakily replied.

As stated previously, Stroke is a great leveller, but there is always somebody, either through breeding or self-perception, that manages to stand out above the common herd. E-bay had Sir Surgical Sock.

An elderly man, who I estimated as to being well in to his nineties, and formerly a surgeon, who certainly had a certain presence about him, and despite a degree of dementia, probably brought on by his stroke, unhesitatingly believed himself entitled to be treated with the respect to which, in his opinion, a man of his professional status should receive. He was very demanding, and my opinion was that when he told the staff to jump, they often did. He would be inclined to bark orders at them and insist on medical procedures that probably were totally irrelevant to his condition. Doctors, nurses, carers and housekeeping staff, all without exception, humoured him and to my mind over-indulged him. However, it must have been difficult for those young people to nurse a surgeon, who had probably retired when they were mere babies or possibly before they were born. They must have been in awe of such a man who had a lifetime of experience in the medical profession. It was quite probable that 'S.S.S' had had a long and distinguished career.

Perhaps I might be accused of being an old scaredy-cat, but I decided that I would certainly shy away from anyone, however eminent, had they expressed the wish to perform surgery on me, especially if they had retired before Fleming had discovered penicillin.

The staff did appear to become sycophantic when tending to the needs of Sir Surgical Sock, but I am sure that they received some compensation by being able to call such a distinguished man by his first name, together with the knowledge that he was totally reliant upon them to help him perform basic bodily functions. The hospital routine spares nobody's dignity, and if your bum needs wiping it gets wiped, however important you think you are.

Chapter 10

When confined to a hospital bed, unlike in the outer world, it is more likely that the private self is inevitably presented, rather than the public face. Therefore, I found it relatively easy to become something of a poor man's philosopher as I was privileged to observe my fellow patients, as well as the staff, in all their guises. I noticed that those with a complaining personality tended to whinge, the worriers diffused worry around them and the grumpy rarely lightened their dark demeanour. Personally, I tried to keep a smile on my face in the belief that it provided encouragement and bonhomie to those around me, though we all had our 'off-days', including me.

One day I had awoken from a relatively good night's sleep, contented and in good spirits, to a ward bustling with activity. I soon gathered, from the countenances of the staff, that they were also somewhat stressed. Sir Surgical Sock was being particularly demanding. He was securing one hundred per cent ministration, which I keenly felt, under the circumstances, was at the expense of other patients, myself included. It seemed that, as an insurance company advertisement used to proclaim, 'Making a Drama out of a Crisis.' paid dividends.

I sat up in my bed, smiling, and attempted a croaky greeting to those that hurried past without a sideways glance. 'The Invisible Man' is not a part that best suits my personality, and I was beginning to convince myself that I *was* invisible. I hailed a nurse, who was a new face to me, as she walked past for the tenth time.

"Good morning" I called, "please stop and make eye-contact, my name is Harold, and I have always found being ignored somewhat off-putting!"

She stopped, mid-stride, as though hit by a sniper's bullet. "Do you realise that you have walked past me ten times without so much as a glance in my direction. I know that you are busy, but it is not good enough. A smile takes up no time at all, but I can assure you, as a patient, that it can be as healing as a spoonful of medicine. I don't suppose that it appears on any of the lists of NHS management targets, but perhaps it should!" I ranted.

"I do not ignore my patients; I am certainly not *that* sort of person!" she retorted defensively.

"I am sure that you are not, but today you have been!" I said crossly.

Her final response was to dissolve into laughter as she disappeared behind the curtains surrounding the bed of Sir Surgical Sock. I sat up in bed, feeling embarrassed, and a little annoyed with myself, that I had allowed my exasperation to surface and quietly dreaded that my outburst might lead me to being put on the 'naughty step'. I was telling myself that I would apologise at the first opportunity when I overheard her say, from behind the curtain, to her colleagues,

"I have just deservedly received a good 'rollicking', in the nicest possible way, from the patient in bed one. Bless him."

It had certainly turned in to a weird morning, to be sure. I'm not superstitious, by nature, but I couldn't help thinking that we must be on the cusp of a full moon.

Dear old 'Awry John', he who cuddled wild rabbits and ignored most advice, voiced his concerns that he had mislaid something important to him and decided to get out of bed to look for it. With an accompanying wail he took a dive worthy of a premiership striker. I immediately pushed my personal alert button in order to summon some emergency assistance for him. This, of course, proved quite unnecessary, as two carers tended to him almost immediately. They picked him up, manoeuvred him back to bed and made him comfortable. He had caused himself no harm and was soon sitting up bolstered by three pillows.

"Here's the mint that I thought I'd lost" he said to himself, with evident satisfaction, as he popped a small, white, sugar coated ball in his mouth, "I do love mints!" The little episode that had resulted in an eddy of mayhem was already forgotten as he sucked, satisfyingly, on the sweet that nearly got away.

Meanwhile, the emergency light above my bed continued to flash, un-noticed apparently, for over thirty minutes. In that period, I was intrigued that nobody had come to ask after my welfare, offered to chaperone me to the toilet, or enquire whether I was in any way troubled. Perhaps it was The Stroke Ward's version of the naughty step!

A staff nurse eventually arrived to administer drugs through the cannula that had been placed in my arm due to my inability to swallow tablets. After my smile was not reciprocated, yet again, I decided to lighten the moment with some idle chat. "It's no fun being fed through this nasal tube when you've got a nose as large as mine. It was nearly three o'clock yesterday afternoon before I tasted my breakfast!" I received a blank stare in return. Whatever, I thought it was funny and laughed enough for the two of us.

On further investigation I ascertained that, due to a management decision, the ward had been left two or three members short of its usual compliment. Of course, this had placed an extra burden and more pressure on a staff, though reduced in number, that were still expected to care for a ward full of very ill patients. It was obvious that there was little time for cosy little chats, especially silly ones.

I was certainly sympathetic, even though the executive decision, had caused a certain amount of collateral damage, as far as the patients were concerned.

I would still have enjoyed a cosy chat, especially with one of those faceless managers.

Chapter 11

One of the downsides of a prolonged stay in hospital is the constant change in personnel. Like in all facets of life, some people are easy to like and others a little more difficult, but the biggest problem is that there is often neither the time nor opportunity to work on relationships. Maybe not too much of a problem to some, but to me, as a patient, I discovered to be very important.

At the commencement of each morning and evening shift, it was probable that we'd be confronted by some new faces. At 'change-over', each team of staff is well informed and drilled about the needs of the individual patients being entrusted to their care. However, there were still, on occasions, breakdowns of communication. This can be frustrating and tiresome for both patients and carers, and from a patient's point of view can negatively impact on morale and confidence.

I suppose one certainty about a stay in hospital is the uncertainty, and initially I found this difficult to get my head around

"You will be home by Friday!"

Three weeks later I am still in bed and now being told,

"You will be having a scan in the morning".

I anticipated that this would most probably take place the following evening. I had learned to take 'fake news' in my stride!

I had also been advised that I would be receiving a visit from a speech and language therapist, so I should not have been surprised when one turned up, but I was!

"Pleased to meet you Harold, my name's Jill and I am the specialist for speech and language. We have been studying your new onset dysphagia, which is the medical term for swallowing difficulties, and your worsening dysphonia which is the term to describe your speaking difficulty. Though still a bit of a mystery, we are convinced that these conditions have not been brought on as the result of you suffering a further event, i.e. another stroke. We would like you to undergo a videofluoroscopy in order to further understand the problems."

"Hang on Jill," I retorted, "I have enough trouble trying to remember the weird and wonderful names of premiership footballers, let alone all this medical terminology. What's a videofluoroscopy?"

Jill proceeded to explain the procedure.

"It is an X-ray that looks at the way your swallowing works. It is one of the tests which can be used to investigate any problems you have with swallowing. It gives a clear picture of what is happening in your mouth and throat when you swallow, and it allows the medical team to see if there are ways to make your swallow safer and easier. You will be seated in front of an X-ray machine and be requested to swallow different kinds of food and drinks of different consistencies. You may find the taste unusual because a contrast, a special liquid that shows up on the X-ray, will be added to the food and drink. As you swallow, we will view what is happening to your mouth and throat. We also make a video recording of the test. There are no tubes involved and it doesn't hurt"

Jill continued to explain that if food goes down the wrong pipe, i.e. the trachea instead of the oesophagus, apart from causing serious choking, it can also enter the lungs causing pneumonia and could eventually prove fatal. The videofluoroscopy would establish exactly what happens when I attempted to swallow. If my swallow was malfunctioning, I would have to continue to be fed by a Nasal Gastric Tube or some other direct method of feeding. I was quietly alarmed when she suggested that this could become my feeding regime for many months or even years to come. The thought of not savouring the taste of sticky toffee pudding ever again rendered me almost suicidal.

Like a genie appearing from a bottle, a hospital porter appeared beside my bed pushing a wheelchair. "Your carriage awaits sir, climb aboard young man! Your presence is required in the X-ray department" he said cheerfully. For him it was just another day at the coal face, yet for me, from what I had just been told by Jill, his routine trip could well herald the greatest ever upheaval in the quality of my life and lifestyle. We chatted amiably as we made our way along the hospital corridors. I was grateful for his friendly manner, as it enabled me to camouflage my nervousness under the veneer of light conversation.

At the department I was met by two speech and language therapists, a radiologist (specialist doctor) and a radiographer, who records the procedure. They put me at ease and then continued the procedure as had been described to me by Jill. I guess I was being X-rayed for approximately half an hour. By turning my head to one side, I managed to swallow small amounts of liquid as well as custard and yoghurt. From the comments of the technicians, I gathered that this was positive. They disappeared behind a glass screen and studied the images that had been taken and viewed the video of my swallow. They commented on their observations to one another. The radiologist dictated her final analysis to her colleagues.

"The images show a moderate oropharyngeal dysphagia characterised by generalised pharyngeal weakness resulting in considerable post swallow residue. Trace penetration was observed with normal fluids. No aspiration was observed. Aerophagia was also found together with backflow and stasis of bolus and a cricopharyngeal spasm."

What had been totally unintelligible was brought starkly in to focus, as she turned to me and said, "Harold, you have a weakness in the muscles that work the epiglottis, but when you do manage to swallow the food flows down your oesophagus and not the windpipe. I recommend that the nasal gastric tube be removed and that you revert to a pre-mashed diet, and I suggest you eat with your head turned to the left so that pharyngeal residue is reduced. We will set you up on some exercises to strengthen your swallow as well as your voice."

Tears of relief welled up in my eyes. If I had had the mobility, I would have jumped from the chair and hugged them all. But, in my head, I slid across the room on my knees as I had regularly watched goal-scorers do in celebration.

"I'm going to get better" I croaked feebly.

By the time I had returned to the ward, news of my results had superseded me. Apart from the minor aberrations, such as cannulas inserted painfully and blood tests taken unnecessarily, the nursing team more than compensate as they cheer each little victory of their patients, like walking to the loo (or should I say shuffling) without too much of a stumble. Now, they genuinely shared my own feelings of relief and happiness that the N.G.T. had been removed.

My little housekeeping friend Mimi appeared with a plate of mashed banana and handed me a fork. "Eat this, 'Aroold, soon 'ave you back on your foot!"

I eased the prongs of the fork under and tentatively lifted a small portion of the mashed fruit. My emotions at that moment can only be described as a joy tinged with fear. The happiness that I was going to taste flavours again was only tempered by the anxiety that I might not be able to swallow. I sucked the banana from the fork and tossed it around my mouth as I summoned up the courage to make my first attempt at a swallow for over ten days. I felt like a high-diver making his first nervous plunge from the ten-metre board. As I had been instructed, I leant my head to the left. I am sure it was more of a gulp than a swallow, but the banana slipped effortlessly down my throat in the correct direction. Not a cough or a wretch, it appeared that I was good at it!

I conjured up a memory of the iconic sports commentator, the late-David Coleman and wondered how he would have described my efforts to the TV viewers.

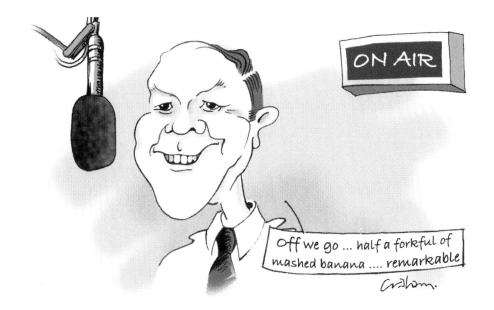

Off we go ... half a forkful of mashed banana .... remarkable

Graham.

"...and off we go...half a forkful of mashed banana has gone straight on to the tongue, he's deftly moved it from the right to the left of his mouth. He's leaning his head over to the left, it's almost resting on his left shoulder. Wow! A massive swallow! The food has gone, his mouth is empty... it's remarkable!!"

Prior to the time when the first evening visitors were anticipated, Jill came to see me again. This time in order to introduce me to a programme of exercises designed to strengthen the muscles that aid swallowing and a further set of exercises to strengthen my voice. I was keen to get started on them.

Never in my wildest dreams would I ever have imagined that the time would come when I would respond so positively to being encouraged to commence pharyngeal strengthening and voice therapy exercises.

When fitness and training routines had been planned for me, over the years, at my local leisure centre, strengthening the voice of Harold Lawrence would most probably have been discouraged! There would probably have been celebrations and dancing in the streets if the news had got out that Harold Lawrence, due to a wonky vocal cord, was now only half as loud!

Times and circumstances change, and I can assure you that when the volume of your speech recedes to hardly an audible croak, a perfect set of biceps, pecs and six packs pale into insignificance against the toning of the muscles attached to the epiglottis and the larynx.

I also felt that it was a tangible step towards my recovery, whilst I also visualised that my attempts at performing the exercises would provide an opportunity to amuse myself and even entertain others.

There were four sets of exercises designed to work and strengthen the pharynx. The first was a chin tuck against the resistance of a sponge ball. The instruction was to press the chin down steadily then control lifting your chin back up to resting position. This had to be repeated thirty times, three times per day. This was followed by 'The Masako' which entailed protruding your tongue between your front teeth and holding it in place by gently biting on the front portion of your tongue then swallowing your saliva. This martial art was performed three times and at least five times per day. Having achieved this, one quickly moved on to the 'Effortful Swallow'. This is effectively the process of swallowing saliva, an interesting development for me, who had, because of the decline in my condition, become a competent exponent of directing my saliva at the spittoon. You imagine that you are trying to swallow a hard golf ball and you use the throat muscles to squeeze the ball down your throat. This is repeated three times at least five times a day. The fourth and one which I found most difficult was 'The Bulldog'. Push the lower jaw forward and whilst maintaining this posture push your tongue up on to your palate, behind your top teeth and swallow your saliva. This also had to be repeated three times and at least five times per day!

That was the 'gurning' lessons taken care of, but now came the voice therapy plan, designed to release tension in the throat. Jill furnished me with another sheet of instructions.

'Take in a deep breath (without letting your shoulders rise). Breathe out on an "extended sssssss" sound; now "zzzzzz"; now "shhhhh"; then "mmmmmm". After this, breathe out on an "extended sssssss" again and then let it change smoothly into an "extended zzzzzz"'

A cautionary note was added:

'Make sure you stop before you run out of air'.

It would be just my luck to have my stroke recovery prematurely halted by a lack of air, I thought.

Provided I had survived part one, I would be able to progress to part two; 'Yawning.' I was optimistic that this might well be an exercise that promised a high degree of success. I have always been a naturally lazy individual, prone to low levels of concentration and becoming effortlessly bored. Yawning had always been one of my strengths, though, come to think of it, it was also perceived as a serious weakness by some of my schoolteachers. I continued to read the instruction.

'This opens up the mouth, exercises the muscles and opens up the jaw. A yawn can also be taken into a body stretch. Lift your arms and stretch to your fingertips, and if sitting, into your legs and toes'.

"This is a new dimension" I thought, "I've always yawned in the past because I couldn't be arsed to do anything else!"

Now for the final part of the Voice Therapy Plan.

'Hum, while blowing through a straw!"

Yes, honestly. I couldn't believe my good fortune. This was an exercise that really appealed to me and transported me back to the days when being the classroom clown was far more enjoyable than trying to get my head round the intricacies of mental arithmetic.

The instructions continued...

'Have a cup with a small amount of water in it and a straw. Take a deep breath in and while breathing out, hum, while blowing through the straw and making bubbles. Try to make the sound continuous and a gentle easy sound, at an easy volume.'

"Easy" I thought.

'It should not feel forced. It is just to warm up the vocal-cords'. (or a cord in my case, apparently). To my knowledge, singing was not encouraged on the ward, but I was optimistic that after a couple of weeks blowing down a straw and humming, I might regenerate the cord that was no longer working and regain the ability to croon myself to sleep.

Chapter 12

I remember viewing the televised Christmas morning visits to Children's wards at various hospitals. Though I obviously felt sorry that they were ill, and unable to be at home with their parents, I was also rather envious of the good time that they seemed to be having. I know the grass is always greener on the other side of the fence, but to a little lad who had just finished emptying a pillowcase containing various little plastic toys, Ludo, Snakes and Ladders, an apple, a tangerine, a Brazil nut and a two bob bit, the presents the children received from Father Christmas, together with the visits from footballers and TV stars, appeared to be a remarkably good deal. Spending time in hospital at Christmas seemed to be and was often spoken about as being great fun. The young patients always appeared happy and cheerful. As a child, myself, I used to think that they, too, felt sorry for those unfortunate children, like me, that had to spend Christmas at home with their parents.

I was still harbouring the belief that spending Christmas in Hospital was only bettered by visiting FC in Lapland. My own common sense should have told me that my fellow residents in the stroke unit were highly unlikely to be jumping out of their beds in order to dance around the Christmas tree. By the way, if they had felt so inclined, they would have been out of luck, as there wasn't one!

Christmas Eve dawned a little late for the housekeeping staff, as they were already, not only demanding menu choices for this day, like any other, but also dishing out the porridge, cornflakes, orange juice, yoghurts and toast. I attempted to introduce a little gaiety to the proceedings by wearing my blue and white 'Seagull's Santa-hat' (The seagulls being the nickname of my football team). I had cultivated a beard over the past month, so I thought it was appropriate to greet the members of staff with a festive "Yoh! Ho! Ho!"

"Porridge...orange juice...mashed banana?" was the deadpan response.

'Hospital Routine' is sacrosanct. The morning's drug round was being dispensed by the busily efficient Frenchman, Soeur Intense. He treated me to a quizzical look and told me that he found it difficult to understand how anybody could get excited about a little team like 'The Seagulls', but PSG (Paris St. Germaine), apparently, was quite a different proposition. I privately doubted that he had ever believed in Father Christmas. Despite not being a believer and his lack of football knowledge, I sincerely hoped that old FC would remember him – as he never fails to put in an energetic shift caring for us patients.

You don't have to be an Einstein to realise that Christmas in a hyper-acute stroke unit is just another day at the office. A Stroke unit is a ward where patients are nursed by a team of highly trained specialists in stroke care. It is thanks to dedicated professionals, such as those on the ward, that there are one point two million stroke survivors in the UK. More people are surviving stroke than ever before. Now, I'm by no means a mathematician, but when one thinks of the number of future Christmases that have been granted to so many stroke patients, thanks to the care and expertise of such gifted people, it would seem extremely churlish to complain about the lack of yule-tide decorations, 'jingle-bells' and other Christmas baubles.

Day dovetailed into evening. The day shift handed over to the night shift. I wondered what type of person would be prepared to work on Christmas Eve, rather than be out partying the night away or attending Midnight Mass. I did not recognise any of the faces, but, whatever their motivation, I for one was grateful for their care.

Like so many things that had happened to me, since being rushed to hospital, I am at a loss to describe my experience of Christmas in hospital other than being as different to any other in my life. There may not have been any glitter balls, balloons, streamers or the noise of corks popping out of bottles of fizzing 'Prosecco', but the ward was far from silent.

Though the lights were dimmed, any encouragement to sleep was dispelled by the general commotion in the workplace. There seemed to be lots of bed removals and conversations between members of staff who seemed not to know each other particularly well. I assumed they were bank staff enticed by an enhanced hourly rate to work unsociable hours. My supposition was soon opened to question as I found myself listening to the following conversation:

"Have you been in the UK for long?"

"Approximately two years."

"Where are you from?"

"I come from a village nearly thirty kilometres from Manila...my family have a small farm. They keep chicken, pigs, grow a little corn. It is very difficult... and you...where are you from?"

"I am West African. My father is the King of our tribe. We are very wealthy. I am in the UK to widen my horizons!"

"Are you a Prince?"

"Well, yes... but it is not something that I would prefer to be widely known. I live modestly and that suits me."

Phew! This was undoubtedly top gossip and with me being, by nature, an inquisitive sort of bloke, I thought it would be too good to miss by carelessly nodding off to sleep. But that is exactly what I did.

Not too many people can boast to having been shaken awake, on Christmas morning, by a member of a Royal Family, masquerading as an NHS Care Assistant.

"Sorry to wake you, Harold, but I need to do your obs."

I do admit to a little disappointment that it wasn't Prince Harry, but I guess he was moonlighting at a different hospital.

It would be wrong to infer that Christmas passed by the Stroke Ward without recognition.

67

An NHS choir, sent on prescription I presumed, robustly and, most importantly, melodiously, sang the carol, 'God Rest Ye Merry Gentlemen', to us recumbent old fellows in E Bay, before hurrying on to the next group of patients.

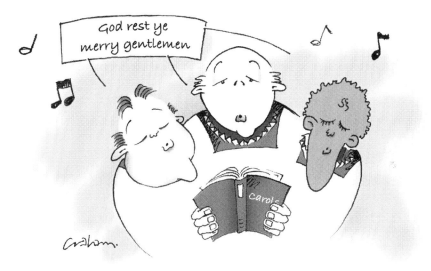

Soeur Intense' stopped by to tell me that the Mayor, accompanied by the Hospital Trust's CEO and other worthies had visited briefly. He said that he had suggested they come and say hello to me, but, had been told that they had a lot to do and wouldn't be stopping. I suggested that that was a poor excuse when one considers how many visits around the world Father Christmas makes in under twenty-four hours. Soeur Intense's face returned a blank look of incomprehension, which to my way of thinking, confirmed, my initial suspicion, that he was a non-believer in Santa. Yet, as if to disprove my theory, he gave me a present and a Christmas-cracker, which were purported to have come from the Man himself!

I impatiently tore the Christmas wrapper off my present, like I used to as a kid, and was delighted with the surprise bottle of hair conditioner. It is heart-warming to know that the few hairs preserved on my head after a balding process, that began in my twenties, would remain vibrant and free of dandruff.

It was a bizarre Christmas. All the family visited, and presents were exchanged but despite the efforts of us all to be upbeat, if I am honest, the celebrations were subdued. I felt extremely guilty. My illness had put untold stress on Angela, the children and the grandchildren. Their Christmas had been disrupted and despite the genuine attempts by us all to exude the Christmas spirit, I admit that, and please excuse the analogy, it was like having an artificial Christmas tree rather than a Nordic spruce.

Visiting time over, I felt rather depressed. The families returned to their respective Christmas Dinners and I was left with an empty feeling in the pit of my stomach. But my brief lapse to self-pity was soon replaced by anticipation of tasting the Christmas Fayre of the NHS.

My imagination conjured up slices of turkey breast with pigs in blankets, sprouts, carrots and golden crispy roast potatoes. I had of course forgotten that I had only stopped being fed through a nasal tube two days before and that I was now restricted to pre-mashed food. Imagine my surprise, therefore, when a small plate containing a pie chart was placed in front of me. There were no written instructions provided but I soon deduced that the grey sector represented turkey, green for the sprouts, orange for carrots and the brown, streaked with black, I supposed was a concoction of spud and chipolata. With some trepidation, I picked up my fork and prodded. As I lifted it, the whole of the contents of the plate adhered itself to the prongs like a multi-coloured cardboard discus.

"Stop, Harold! you can't eat that!"

Dear 'Soeur Intense' was, in his own fashion, again presenting a caring face to the world. I could not help but recall the story about Sir Walter Raleigh when he was said to have thrown his cloak over a puddle to save his Sovereign from getting her feet wet. On this occasion, I was the grateful recipient of a similar selfless act of consideration.

69

Soeur Intense snatched away my pie chart, and a few short minutes later replaced it with a plate of mashed cod in a white sauce. Not the feast of Turkey and Pudding that I had contemplated, but very tasty none the less and much appreciated.

Christmas day drifted to its conclusion with the day shift again replaced by the night-time operatives. Having learned nothing from previous experience, I made the mistake of becoming complacent and feeling 'at home' and well looked after in E-bay. I had said a fond 'Au Revoir' to the carers and had told them how much I was looking forward to seeing them all again on Boxing Day.

Obviously the 'Powers that Be' were unimpressed with too much fraternisation, and thirty minutes into Boxing Day, I was awoken from a light sleep to be told that I was being moved from E-bay into a general ward. I was advised that there were four, recently arrived, stroke patients languishing in A&E who were urgently waiting for beds to become available.

It would have seemed selfish to have complained, even though my removal was rather undignified. The contents of my bedside locker were unceremoniously piled on top of my bed together with my dressing gown, slippers and walking frame. I felt like a victim of an avalanche. Pinned to the mattress, with just one free arm that allowed me to wave goodbye to Grumpy Mal, and Allawry John, who had both been disturbed and woken by the commotion.

My bed was pushed, by a burly porter, through the portals of E-bay for the last time.

Chapter 13

After a relatively short time, I was surprised by the extent that I had assumed the role of a permanent resident of the Stroke ward. So much so that, on completion of my move, I felt like a displaced person. Removal to a new ward was not unlike entering the hospital system for the first time. There was a definite need to rewind the mental clock. With new staff, and new faces, I was confronted, again, with the need to broker new relationships. I had been advised that the ward predominantly treated cardiac and diabetes patients, though approximately fifty per cent of the present incumbents were stroke patients, who like me, had been transferred in, due to the urgent need for beds in the acute stroke ward. It provided me, yet again, a stark reminder that a large percentage of the population in the UK, from all age groups, suffer this serious breakdown in their health.

I know that I have already grumbled about this, but as my stay in hospital lengthened, I had no reason to alter my opinion that the system sometimes showed up a distinct lack of continuity.

Too often, there was a need to explain to new carers the rules, that have been previously laid down for you by their colleagues elsewhere. As a patient, there were times when I found this an exasperating and frustrating necessity. Although I am sure it was not so, I sometimes gained the impression that 'modus operandi' notes were being jealously protected by their authors, instead of being passed on to the next point of patient contact.

This, along with the lack of certainty, from day to day, were the things that I found the most difficult to get my head around, and I learned to take, with a pinch of salt, authoritative statements such as "You will be going home by Friday." Even after twenty-two days and three wards later, I was still unsure which Friday they were talking about.

I was assured that all my treatments would continue, as scheduled, yet I could not restrain a nagging doubt that I was about to experience a side of the NHS that had become grist to the media mill.

I sensed that the ethos in this ward was completely different from the one I had been removed. This realisation unnerved me slightly. My bed had been placed next to a window, but any prospect of a view was hampered by towels that had been strategically placed to soak up the ingress of water entering through the gaps in the ill-fitting window frame. I felt a distinct draught which reminded me, for the first time in nearly a month, that the world outside was still languishing in winter.

I was now being confronted with the effects of an under-resourced NHS during a critical winter period. I now began to comprehend why it had become the cornerstone of media interest. The many timely warnings and cries of help, from all grades of the medical profession, had been ignored. We now had to put up with much huffing, puffing, frothing and excusing from politicians in reaction to the reality of the situation. After all, had it not even provoked a noble Lord to resign from his role as an NHS hospital trustee?

I realised that up to now I had been the recipient of the best of care that the NHS provides. From the time of admission, I had been cared for by professionals, specifically trained in the care and recovery of stroke patients. My previous wards provided both hyper-acute and acute stroke care. Doctors work alongside a dedicated nursing team and are supported by neuro-physiotherapists, dieticians, occupational therapists and speech and language therapists. It was one of the largest of such units in the UK and was very highly rated. Yes, it was truly a flagship of the Hospital Trust.

My new-found circumstances brought to my mind the clichés Chalk and cheese and feast and famine. It was plaintively clear to me that there was a big discrepancy in the ratio of the number of carers to patients, and that the additional workload and stress that was imposed upon the caring staff was quite often reflected on their countenances. This is certainly not a criticism of them, but rather on a system that is sustained by imposing busy, stressful twelve hour shifts upon individuals.

Though still sharing a bay with five other patients, and only a hundred yards away from my former ward, I felt very lonely and unashamedly sorry for myself. I certainly missed 'Grumpy Mal' and his temper tantrum that he always displayed to the unfortunate nurse who, on 'Obs' patrol, was designated to wake him in the morning. I'm sure that his blood pressure was always high and equally sure, that it returned to normal once he had had his breakfast and calmed down! I also missed listening to Awry John's unwavering contention that the Hospital authorities planned to kill us all by radiation, and I admit that I rather liked the confident presence of Sir Surgical Sock constantly demanding and expecting that the staff should respect 'yesterday's man' and accordingly pay him obeisance.

"So, there you are!"

For the second time during my stay in hospital, I was shaken from a maudlin moment by a familiar and unexpected voice.

"Mal! What are you doing here?"

There was a certain amount of déjà vu about this conversation. Pyjama clad, Mal made long strides towards me down the middle of the bay holding aloft his walking frame. I could tell from the faces of my mystified fellow patients that they were convinced this stranger was about to use his surgical appliance as a weapon to beat me over the head. Of course, they were unaware it was Mal being Mal and refusing to be told that he needed assistance of any sort. After all, weren't these carers just watching their own backs?

"It's Health and Safety gone mad – that's the trouble with this country!" Mal would say.

Two more strides and then Mal fell headlong across my bed.

"Oops!" he said, "I hope the secret police didn't see that!"

"Pull up a bed, why don't you?" I said. "Don't worry about anyone seeing your acrobatics, Mal, this isn't the Stroke Ward, they haven't got enough people here with time to waste on rule-breakers."

"It was carrying that flipping walking frame that made me lose my balance." said Mal, steadfastly refusing to accept that he might be in any way responsible for the mishap.

"Perhaps carrying it does cause a problem." I sympathised, "Surely the nurses should have thought of that. Flipping Health and Safety!"

I was truly pleased that Mal had taken the trouble and the risk to pay me a visit. It certainly cheered me up.

"Do they know that you have come to visit me?"

"No, I just fancied a stroll and one of the Household staff told me that you had been moved to here, which I guessed would be close by, and so here I am!"

"Good to see you mate. But you had better make it back because you are sure to have been missed. I think I heard the Lifeboat maroons go off just now and there is definitely the sound of a chopper overhead."

Mal started to walk away. Then he stopped, turned his head towards me, and displayed the hint of a grin.

"You are a silly sod!"

He was a good bloke, Mal. He really didn't set out to be difficult, but he just had a bit of a problem with Authority, that he had clearly honed, to an art form, over the past seventy years or so.

Mal's unexpected arrival and departure served to reinforce a worry that had been festering within me since I had been in this new ward. An apparent lack of supervision encouraged in me an irrational feeling that I had been abandoned.

I filled in the quiet moments by indulging in the pastime of 'people –watching'.

In the bed opposite was a chap called Bill, a stroke patient, probably in his late forties, who seemed to have been left with numerous disabilities.

Bill's wife had told my wife, during a visiting-time, that he was suffering from Aspasia, had a problem with swallowing, and paralysis down the right side of his body which caused him great difficulty in walking, even with the aid of a walking frame. I was astonished and full of admiration at the way he managed to cope, with the minimum of assistance. He was obviously a determined and independent bloke. I am quite sure that he preferred to get on with his life with the minimum of fuss.

However, I am equally sure that he would never have got away with it in The Stroke Ward, where I had personally been instructed not to take a single step without somebody accompanying me. In this ward, I noted, there seemed to be no such inhibitions.

In the bed next to Bill was Mr. Patel, who had, apparently, been waiting since yesterday for a transfer to another hospital. His wife sat patiently beside him as they waited for the logistics to be finalised. There was a flurry of activity when two nurses turned up by his bed, one of whom was carrying a sheaf of papers.

"This was it!" I thought, "Mr. Patel is on the move, after God knows how many hours of waiting!"

But no. I overheard him being asked to complete a dreaded NHS survey form. How is it *they* always managed to arrive on time?

If you have never been asked to complete one of these, you are probably rude in health and never been even close to any of the NHS establishments.

It seems to me that the management have a neurotic obsession to seek feed-back from patients at every opportunity. All departments throughout the NHS request patients to complete these questionnaires and place their responses in a little post box which, I have noticed, are emptied regularly by a 'post person'.

My belief is, that when things go well, grateful patients are only too happy to tell them. However, when things go wrong, I am sure that a complainant would be unlikely to express his or her feelings by answering a factitious question, on a scrap of paper. Then patiently wait for the NHS's response.

I recalled the time, when I was in extreme pain, suffering from kidney stones. I was laying on a treatment table in A&E, waiting for the doctor to give me the results of a scan, along with her diagnosis. A young nursing-assistant arrived holding a piece of paper, which she handed to me, together with a ball-point pen.

"Please complete this before leaving", she said, abruptly, before walking away.

Of course, it was a survey form. Unless she intended to find out how many expletives that I could fit on to a ten-centimetre line, the young nurse had been way off from choosing the right psychological moment. I decided that it would be prudent to put it in to my pocket and leave the form-filling to a time when I was feeling a lot better and able to concentrate.

By the way, I got around to completing the form, some days later. I confess that I had forgotten its existence until I came across it, when emptying my jacket pockets. I gave it a cursory glance.

"Please respond to the questions by circling a number. 1-10, where number I0 is definitely; Number1 is not bloody likely (or words to that effect.)

Question one – "Would you recommend us to your friends and family?"

I wonder who thought that one up? I had been in the A&E Department, after all.

I scratched my head. Was there an alternative service that could be recommended? I Imagined myself coming across the victim of an accident, lying in the middle of the road after being knocked up in the air by a motor car. How would I deal with the situation?

"Keep calm, old chap, I will send for an ambulance or alternatively, I could send for the 'Medicines San Frontiere'. I have been told that they are excellent in an emergency. Unfortunately, it is likely that you may have to stay where you are for a day or two as they are busy in Africa."

Come on! Wake up and smell the coffee, Mr/Mrs/Miss Survey Designer.

Mr. Patel, said that he would have great difficulty complying with this, request. But he was not to be excused, as this exercise was obviously an essential and important step towards his eventual recovery. A compromise was agreed. The questions would be read to him by one of the nurses and his answers would be written down for him by the other... I was totally intrigued by this evolving little play. Sadly, for me, this was as close as I was going to get to entertainment!

"Question number one." said nurse one, "On a scale of one to four, one being definitely, four being not at all, would you recommend this ward to your friends and family?"

"Yes-one" said Mr. Patel, with a smile and a twinkle in his eye.

"Question number two—on the same scale, one being excellent, four very poor, what do you consider the quality of treatment that you have received in the General Ward?

"Yes—one" responded Mr. Patel, without hesitation.

"Question number three-same scale, what is your opinion of the menu and quality of meals?"

"One-the food has been wonderful"

"Finally, is there any area of your treatment which you feel could have been improved?"

"No."

From my bed, I assumed the role of a judge, the likes of whom might be seen on Strictly Come Dancing or the X Factor, and called out that in my humble opinion Mr. Patel had scored 'a ten' proving to the world that he was a very astute man, and had earned his passage through to the next stage of his recovery. Mrs P. Smiled, and Mr. P gave me a little wave of acknowledgement followed with a thumbs up. The two nurses, however, by the look on their faces, were not so impressed by my efforts to lighten the moment.

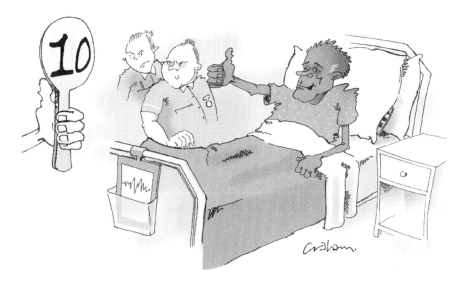

Had the two of them been more personable, they might, perhaps, have provided an answer to a question that was bouncing around in my brain.

How had Mr. Patel managed to secure the services of two nurses in order to complete a survey, when I hadn't set eyes on anybody since being disturbed from my semi-consciousness state at the dawning of day shift?

"Good morning gentlemen. My name is Grace, and I will be looking after you today. If you need me, just call…"

Grace had kept to the NHS 'early morning introduction' script, which to my mind, and in in fairness to all the carers and patients, should have concluded with these additional words...

"... unfortunately, I will subsequently be kept so busy that it is likely that I will rarely be seen again by you. Please accept my apologies in advance, but that's how the system works!"

Despite my strong desire to be a latter-day Che Guevara and lead a patients' revolt within this small corner of the NHS, I do confess that neither my question nor my suggested improvement to Grace's script were ever put.

To my shame, I confess that the conventionalist within me bottled it!

Chapter 14

The Oxford English Dictionary defines flotsam as wreckage from a ship found floating. I could not help feeling that this, after twenty-four days as a guest of the NHS, was my newly acquired patient-status in in the General Ward. I formed the impression that they had taken stroke-survivor Harold Lawrence as far as they could and were now seeking the earliest opportunity to move him on to more appropriate care elsewhere.

I may have become over-sensitive, but I was convinced that somewhere in the bowels of the Hospital, there was a committee of anonymous administrators discussing the fate of NHS Patient, number 001 437 7777.

Blimey, I had progressed to be a stroke survivor with paranoia!

"How will they entertain me today?" I wondered. "I'll ask Grace, about the itinerary."

Of course, she wouldn't know but she will professionally placate my concerns and promise to find out. I will take the opportunity to thank her profusely, as it will probably be the only occasion that I will see her throughout the rest of her long shift.

As the 'flotsam' drifted along with the day, I was pleasantly surprised by a visit from a lady doctor. She was very attractive, sartorially resplendent, and had a personality to match. Half a century ago, I would have fallen head-long in love and tried out all the callow chat-up lines of youth. In the present circumstances, it would have to be of the utmost foolishness to suggest that either I, or she, really cared one iota. Anyway, it was fair to say that I completely lacked either the will, the wit or the 'six-pack' to qualify as anything close to feeling macho.

She advised me that I was, later that day, to expect further blood tests plus a visit from an ENT (Ear, Nose and Throat, apparently) therapist. Though I am sure her plans were properly documented, in what I now assumed was NHS procedure, it followed that none of her plans for me transpired.

Shortly after, I needed to attend to an urgent call of nature. I managed to attract the attention of a nurse and asked her to accompany me to the bathroom. She appeared a little surprised by my request. I was only trying to keep to the procedure strictly enforced by the nursing team in the Stroke Ward. I had been clearly told that I was not to attempt to walk anywhere unless accompanied by a Carer. My health had improved considerably, but I was still very wobbly on my pins and liable to bouts of vertigo. Also, I had become so reliant on others, in the time I had spent in hospital, that my confidence to carry out tasks, independently, had clearly eroded. Although I suspected a lack of comprehension of my situation, she nevertheless followed behind. I did note that it was at a distance which I doubted would have provided me with the safety net that I had been seeking. On arrival, she opened the door to the bathroom and turned back, leaving me to my own devices.

"Give a ring when you have finished" she said over her shoulder, as she closed the door.

I finished, I rang, I waited... and waited and waited and rang again. Fifteen minutes... still no response. There was a rattling at the door handle.

"At last!", I thought, as I manoeuvred myself on the walking frame and opened the door.

To my surprise, it was Bill. I let him in and we both smiled and nodded. I pushed past him and set-off, one slow push of the walking frame followed by a tentative step, laboriously repeated as I retraced my way back to my bed. There was not so much as a glance in my direction from any of the busy staff, when I staggered into and ricocheted off the wall as I passed the nursing station.

Once safely returned, I reconsidered the situation. Bill was far more disabled by his stroke than me, and it seemed, as a casual observer, that there was little concern shown for his safety, by either himself or the ward staff, when he coped on his own. I reasoned, therefore, that from now on, I should not expect to receive any special attention either.

I recalled, as a child, the fun that me and my chums used to have, removing the lids of two cocoa tins and joining both with a length of string to make a telephone. To us it was almost magical that what was said in to one end could clearly be heard at the other. We were convinced that if only we could lay our hands on a long- enough piece of string we would be able to talk to someone in America! Martin Perkins, better known as Prof' by us lesser mortals, possessed knowledge way in excess of the average ten-year-old way back in 1952. He had poured scorn on our careless talk and childish innovation by pointing out, with disdain, that the first transatlantic telephone conversation had already taken place on the 6th January 1927 between two unknown men who talked about the weather. I well remember, defensively countering that our method would be cheaper and that our conversation would be far more interesting. The cowboy, Roy Rogers and 'Champion the Wonder Horse' were two of the suggested subjects.

Whatever the pros and cons, at that moment in time, nothing would convince me otherwise that our attempts at communication, then, still seemed superior and more effective than the alarm bell system currently employed in the Ward.

As inevitable as the ebbing tide, the outside world moved from daylight to darkness. Within the hospital, however, time is governed by routine rather than the position of the sun.

The day shift was imperceptibly replaced by the night shift, and eventually the lights were dimmed, signifying, to the patients, that it was time for sleep. Like the flotsam that I believed I had become, I anticipated drifting through yet another long night. Intermittently dozing between OBS patrols, and the inevitable disturbances caused by busy people tending to the needs of the ill people, until the inevitable wake-up welcome from Nurse Grace or Fritz or whoever else was on the rota to look after us during the day ahead.

I suspect it was because the Ward was deprived of the sophisticated communication equipment that was available to me in my youth, that I had received no hint that this was to be my last night spent in the District Hospital. On reflection, it was probably for the best. If I had suddenly received such seismic news from a faceless person at the other end of the string, I would have been too excited to remember to ask for a weather forecast.

Chapter 15

'When Irish eyes are smiling, you'll be smiling too...' These words from the song were brought back to my mind, on this, the twenty-fifth day after having a stroke.

"Good morning Harold, I am Sister Sean O'Rourke." To my ears, the words flowed in a brogue that was as soft as the waters from the Wicklow Mountains.

For some reason, his name made me think of "Rourke's Drift", the epic film starring Michael Caine about the Zulu Wars. I drew an analogy clearly in my head. Like Michael Caine's character in the film, Sister Sean lead a small band under siege, and, I felt as if I was now, shoulder to shoulder, with them.

"I have some good news for you. You will be going home later today. We just need to complete the paperwork and arrange the pharmacy to stock you up with pills and potions. I understand that you will be needing an extra walking frame too. I will phone your wife and she can come and pick you up."

I was, of course, overjoyed at the prospect but I immediately detected a flaw in the good Sister's planning strategy. I knew how to get four elephants into a Mini – two in the front and two in the back- but how do you get a wobbly bloke, two walking frames, a large bag of medicines and a holdall full of clothes and other personal effects into a Citroen C1?

He was unabashed.

"Have you not got a bigger car between you?"

"Yes, but my wife won't drive it."

"Then, I'll have to arrange some transport which will mean that you won't be able to go home until this afternoon. In the meantime, I will organise a porter to take you down to the Discharge Lounge and the ambulance will pick you up from there"

It was all very reassuring, yet something in my water was telling me that there may be trouble ahead.

I washed, dressed and an hour or two later was sitting in the armchair beside the bed waiting for the moment when the 'Great Escape' would start to materialise. I say 'the' rather than 'my' bed because almost as soon as Sister O'Rourke had gone off to make all the arrangements, two care assistants arrived and stripped away all the bed linen and replaced with fresh, signalling to me that a new patient was imminently expected to take my place.

Visiting time was at 2.00 p.m. Five minutes before, someone from the pharmacy department turned up with two huge bags full of drugs together with a comprehensive list of instructions. How many pills were to be taken at what time of the day and night etc. etc. He also gave me another walking frame, "one for upstairs and one for down, apparently." he said, and left as quickly as he had arrived.

I remained sitting in the armchair, virtually obscured by my newly acquired baggage which had been added to the holdall of clothes and personal effects, outdoor-coat, scarf and gloves. My head felt as if it was poking out of a pile of debris and I was afraid that I would not be found and thus be stuck in hospital for the rest of my life. My fears were unfounded, of course, because hot on the tail of the pharmacist came a porter pushing a wheelchair.

He wasn't too communicative, but I could tell from his demeanour, as he eyed-up me, the baggage and the walking frames, that he was mystified by how he was going to get a quart in a pint pot or a bag lady in a small wheelbarrow.

He scratched his head, and said, I am not sure whether it was to himself or he was addressing me, "Going down to the Discharge Lounge."

Whenever I have attempted to construct an item of furniture or a domestic appliance from a flat-pack, I always manage to have a couple of screws left over! My wife always berates me for not having read the instructions. As a bloke, reading pages of notes goes against the grain. Firstly, it's boring, and secondly, it suffocates the sense of adventure.

I sensed that there was a hint of this syndrome in the porter's actions. He helped me on to the wheelchair and heaped the baggage on top of me. Through a peephole, which I think had been left on purpose, either to allow me to look out or to breathe, I noticed that there were two walking frames left over.

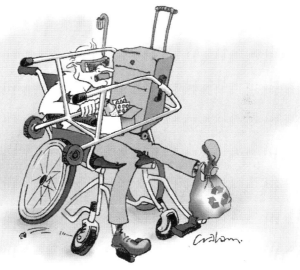

"How are you going to carry them?"

Again, I was not sure to whom he was talking, but in a spirit of self-protection, I called out from the depths, "It's your problem, mate!"

Though I had not heard bugles or the galloping of hooves, at that precise moment the cavalry certainly arrived in the guise of my nephew and niece, Andrew and Annette. They wouldn't have had the slightest idea that their quick visit to see Uncle Harold in hospital would become such a fortuitous event for the patient or the carer. I'm not sure who was the most delighted by their unexpected arrival, me or the porter, but in no time at all they were volunteered to carry a walking frame each and I was purposefully pushed in the direction of the Discharge Lounge. Without realising it, A&A had become a Rescue Service.

In my imagination I had pictured the Discharge Lounge as resembling a Departure Lounge that one might use at Gatwick Airport, with coffee and soft drinks on tap and a finger buffet temptingly stocked to quell the hunger pangs. Reality soon kicked in on arrival. I don't think that I could be accused of over-exaggeration if I described the room as unwelcoming. It had a bed in one corner, an armchair, two hard-backed waiting room chairs and a coffee table that was shouting out for a French polisher or better still a bonfire.

Having parked me by the coffee table, the Porter strolled over to a desk where two frowning nurses were sitting and watching our arrival. They seemed to be guarding the room like a couple of bouncers that might be encountered outside Mirabelle's, and apparently, they were every bit as difficult to get past.

It was made quite clear to the Porter that they didn't know who I was and that they were not expecting anybody transferring from General Ward. The porter shrugged, he'd done what he had been asked to do and it was no longer his problem. Without a backward glance, he trolled off, leaving me in 'no man's land'.

I noticed a hint of panic in the eyes of Andrew and Annette. A well- intentioned short stay beside the hospital bed of their old uncle had somehow escalated into the role of official carers for their very own stroke patient.

Apparently, though not unexpectedly from my point of view, the Ward had not, after all, followed procedure and completed the necessary paperwork that logged me in or out. Urgent telephone calls were made, voices were raised, and I sat in my wheelchair as they endeavoured to prove that patient number 001 437 7777, not only existed but was sufficiently well enough to be sent home.

Twenty minutes later, the computer slowly printed out the required papers, probably in triplicate. After a speedy perusal, one of the nurses sighed, arched her eyebrows and addressed me and the two A's. in a tone that seemed to place the blame for the confusion directly on our doorstep.

"Well, 'problem', despite everything, we have at last established that you should actually be here and that you are to be discharged. Now I have got to arrange some transport for you. If I had been advised earlier, we'd have had a vehicle waiting, but I'm not a mind reader and we are very busy so I expect you will be here for about five hours!"

Yet again, I believed I could read the minds of my visitors.

"Ruddy hell, we're stuck with the old boy for another five hours, we can't leave him…how do we get out of this one?"

I anticipated that they might have made an excuse to go to the toilet and escape through a window. I would have, but they didn't. Obviously much nicer people than me!

We settled into a frame of mind that would fill in the hours ahead with small talk liberally punctuated with silly jokes, which is a family strength or weakness depending on one's point of view.

After barely fifteen minutes, an ambulanceman came into the room. I called out, putting on a silly voice that imitated Spike Milligan.

"'Arold's over 'ere, mate!"

To my utter surprise, he replied, "You're the very man I'm looking for!"

Apparently, Andy, as he introduced himself, and his colleague had earlier in the day transported a patient to one of the London hospitals, expecting to stay there all day. However, they were not required and had made their way back and called in, on the off chance, to see if anyone was waiting for transport. How lucky was I, and what a great relief for A&A!

There were smiles and handshakes all round. 'Arold and baggage were stowed aboard the ambulance. After cheery farewells, we were 'on the road'. I'll soon be home again.

Hurrah!

Chapter 16

Our house is an 'upside-down' property. The bathroom and bedrooms are downstairs with the reception rooms and kitchen upstairs. Andy the ambulance driver, however, had delivered me to a house that had been transformed in to one 'fit for purpose'. By that, I mean, it now contained additional fixtures and fittings designed to aid a wobbly bloke, who now required the aid of walking frames and a wheelchair to get about and function within its walls.

The place had been furnished with perching stools, strategically placed, in the hallway, kitchen and shower. A second bannister had been fitted to the opposite wall on the staircase, the toilet seat had been raised by the fitting of a plastic seat, a commode was introduced upstairs, just in case of an emergency, as we have only got the one bathroom. Besides a wheelchair, I was now the keeper of three NHS walking frames. One to get me to the top of the stairs, one at the bottom of the stairs, to get me in to the bedrooms and bathroom, and a narrower one that would enable me to get in the kitchen. I was grateful for these accoutrements, but it was like having too many unwanted guests sharing your living space. I felt like a stranger in my own, overcrowded, home.

It dawned on me, also, that my extended stay in hospital had institutionalised me to a degree that effected my confidence and I started to worry about how Angela and I would cope with my regained independence and the next chapter of my recovery. It is quite remarkable how soon one slips in to the habit of abdicating the responsibility of day-to-day living to others. I was now passing this mantle, shared by the nursing staff of the District Hospital, on to the shoulders of Angela. Even though I knew that she would suffocate me with care, I was conscious of the huge burden, certainly in the short term, that I was going to be.

Over the next eight weeks Angela's burden was shared magnificently, with professionalism and humour, by the local NHS Community team.

I was cared-for by six wonderful ladies, and in a short time we both looked upon them as friends, and we always anticipated their visits with pleasure. I was a bit of a 'know-all' patient and had plenty to say, but they exhibited great patience and were not slow in telling me my fortune when necessary! Also, I was soon to learn that they looked upon Angela as a team member. In their eyes, she was the only person in the house who possessed the common-sense to keep my nose to the recovery grindstone. I was not offended and agreed with them totally.

My swallowing, diet, talking, balancing and walking were all impaired and needed working on. I still had a numbness down the right-side of my face, and the left side of my body hadn't got much of a clue when it came to the sensations of hot and cold.

A book written by Dale Carnegie crossed my mind. 'The Power of Positive Thinking'. I was having to learn techniques and exercise routines that would re-wire my brain and re-oil the physical mechanisms. I admit that, initially, the challenges that I was being presented with seemed like bridges too far. However, all these wonderful ladies in my life were not only teaching me, but also encouraging me, and could always be relied upon to make a great fuss over every bit of progress made, however minute.

I have always been a person who would try to run before learning to walk and my inherent impatience was exacerbated by my disability. On a scale of one to five, my ability to adjust to invalidity was minus one. For example, I never fully understood the instructions, plainly explained, on how to use a walking frame. You push the frame forward a foot and then walk into it, push the frame forward again, walk into it and thus one slowly makes progress.

"Slow down, Harold! You're not in a go-kart, you're on a Zimmer. Cut out the handbrake turns as well!" was an oft' repeated plea of the physios.

Once I had convinced them that I would not be breaking my neck, I progressed to walking across the room on two walking sticks. But I wasn't too happy.

"They make me feel like an old man. I'd rather use Nordic poles."

This caused a certain amount of controversy between the carers. In fact, there was a fifty-fifty split. The pro-walking stick faction assured me that I would soon get used to walking sticks and they would be safer. The one person who backed my idea was the physio, who was a champion triathlon athlete. With her support, I had my own way and purchased a pair of walking poles. These proved to be a vast improvement. I was walking with an upright posture and they proved to be more efficient in balancing me when the inevitable wobble occurred.

I was delighted, some time afterwards, to be told, thanks to my progress with the poles, they had been recommended to other patients!

A red-letter day arrived when my carers decided they were sufficiently satisfied with my walking, that it was time for me to display my ambulant prowess to the outside world.

It was a great event. Angela waved me goodbye from the front door, as with the aid of my walking poles, and the close attendance of my physiotherapist, along with her colleague, either side of me in case I should fall, I battled up the steep drive from the house. Following, a little way behind, came another carer, pushing a wheelchair. We were like a mini version of the town carnival procession and there was much gaiety in the air as we revellers set off. The world was my oyster, and I was determined to have a successful ramble.

It was decided that we would attempt to walk around the block. The route comprised of two flat stretches, one short but steep incline, and a similar gradient downhill. In total it was over a quarter of a mile. I got into my stride. Pushing on my poles, I felt like a latter-day Captain Scott facing the challenge of crossing the Antarctic. A slight exaggeration, I suppose, but walking down the Lane, up the Avenue, along the Drive and back to the Lane was, in my mind, an equally challenging expedition.

"Slow down, Harold!" called Julie, who was pushing the empty wheelchair.

I waited for her at the top of the incline. I realised that pushing, a wheelchair up a steep slope is no easy task, and as she stopped behind me, her breath was being emitted in short bursts.

"Blimey, Julie, I'm fitter than you!" I said cheekily.

The metamorphosis from winter in to spring reflected the progress of my recovery. The appearance of the first crocus always takes me by surprise. I was similarly surprised, as well as intrigued by the imperceptible progress that I was achieving physically and mentally. How the brain rewires itself is still a mystery to me, but it does happen. It was strange how others had to point out my progress rather than it being noticed by myself. I was bemoaning the slowness of my recovery, whilst those around me were apparently delighted by the speed of it.

Chapter 17

I had set myself goals to reach in the year ahead, and I was determined to achieve them.

My first was to take the Chair, as President, at the AGM and Presentation event of the Disability Football Club which was set for the beginning of April. I had done this for the past fifteen years, and I was determined to prove that there was life after stroke! All our footballers are inspirational people, themselves, who meet and overcome challenges every day of their lives. They will all be there, so me turning up would be hardly exceptional.

I think there was some trepidation mixed in with the encouragement that I received from the Club Committee. I suspect they were concerned by the prospect of having to administer the 'kiss of life' to the President, halfway through the proceedings.

I made it to the event, and all went well. The only clue to my recent predicament were the Nordic poles that were still required to balance me when I got up to speak!

I made a promise to my grandson, Jem, whilst I was still in hospital, that I would get better in time to take him to watch 'The Seagulls' play the mighty Manchester United. This was at the beginning of May, and at the time it seemed many months away. With hindsight, this could have been proven over-optimistic, but the possibility of breaking my promise to him never entered my head.

The great day arrived. It hadn't occurred to me that I would find being part of a thirty thousand crowd so scary. The noise, the pushing and shoving, the need to negotiate a path through crowds of surging people is to be expected, and I hadn't previously thought too much about it. After all, this all added to the flavour and excitement of attending a big game. But post-stroke, with the brain still in the process of re-wiring, it all took a bit of coping with. My walking poles, once again, were useful in helping to create a bit of space around me, but, even then, I was having to suppress surges of panic. My overwhelming sense of responsibility for my grandson, overcame my own fears, so I didn't let on. I dredged up the memory of being a student at 'The Outward-Bound Mountain School' in Eskdale, nearly sixty years ago! The OBMS motto is 'To serve, to strive, but not to yield'. This mantra resonated through my head as I wobbled my way, successfully, to my seat.

Against most supporters' expectations, the Seagulls beat the mighty United by one goal to nil,

All was well, until the Seagulls scored the unexpected winning goal. In the moment, my need of Nordic poles was completely forgotten. As I leapt to my feet, in excitement, I propelled myself over the heads of the row in front. At that precise moment of lift-off, the man sitting next to me grabbed my arm, whilst apologising profusely. He thought that he had knocked me flying as he too had jumped to his feet. I accepted his apology gracefully, after all these things happen, don't they?

My next goal was to resume driving.

Not by any stretch of the imagination could I be labelled a 'petrol-head'. I have never felt sentimental enough about a car to ever attempt to humanise it. I have friends that refer to their cars as "She's a good old girl" and then boast about how much 'she' can do to the gallon. I've never understood how anyone can be seduced by a lump of metal with a wheel at each corner. Yet, when stuck indoors on a walking frame, I used to look out of the window at the driveway on which my car was parked, and it became a symbol of what was once my active life.

"Would I ever drive again?"

I was now gaining a little more independence. With the aid of my Nordic poles, I was walking a couple of miles each day. I was diligently working at the exercises, set me by the physiotherapist, to improve my balance and co-ordination.

Angela drove me, here and there when it was necessary, and I was gradually accepting the role of front-seat passenger. I was poor, however, at supressing my frustration at not being the driver, and poor Angela had to bear the brunt of my grumbles. I appreciated being driven, but for the sake of domestic harmony, I decided to make a positive attempt to regain my driver status by volunteering for a Driving Assessment.

I applied, to South East Driveability for assessment.

I did not have to wait long for an appointment, and I was driven to their centre by my son-in-law, Mark. It was a journey of over thirty miles, and the closer we got, the more nervous I became. I babbled on about probably failing as I calculated that the last time that I had had a driving test was nearly sixty years ago! But as Mark succinctly put it, "So what!"

An Occupational Therapist, and the Driving Assessor, introduced themselves. The assessment was more comprehensive than I had envisaged, and they explained that I would be assessed, not only on my driving, but my physical, cognitive and visual abilities. I was put through a lot of tests, and then asked to drive a Vauxhall Corsa, which was fitted with dual controls. The Assessor sat beside me, giving me directions, whilst the Occupational Therapist sat behind, taking notes. I drove for forty-five minutes around Kent. It was the first time I had driven a car for six months. The traffic was heavy, and not knowing the area at all well, I really had to concentrate.

By the time I returned to the centre I was 'cream-crackered.' I am sure that my brain had been through the process of re-wiring to such an extent that anyone touching my head would have received an electric shock!

The total assessment had taken from 1.30 pm through to 5.00 pm. After a short de-briefing, I was grateful to return to Mark and anxious to get home. I don't remember having much of a conversation with Mark on the return journey, unless I was talking in my sleep.

Two weeks later an A4 size envelope dropped on to the door mat. It contained a seven page 'Driving Assessment Report'. The last time that the butterflies in my tummy were so active was when I received my GCE results. On that occasion I had failed more than I had passed, could this letter signal the end of my driving career?

I started to read.

'Mr Lawrence's speech and language were clear and effective. He was able to hold a coherent conversation with the assessment team and make his needs known'

Well that was a good start. I had been so nervous, that I could have been totally unintelligible. I continued reading

'Mr Lawrence was able to recall the date, month and year during the initial assessment '

Blimey, this brain-rewiring really does work. I could never remember the day of the week even before I had the stroke.

There were seven pages of comment. No stone regarding my driving and mental ability was left unturned. Eventually I could not put off reading the section 'Overall Conclusion & Recommendations' any longer...

'Based upon the evidence gathered on the day of assessment, the team have no hesitation in reporting that Mr Lawrence is currently safe to drive. This was a safe and confident drive today.'

Hallelujah! Perhaps I'm a petrol-head after all. I can't wait to get the old girl back on the road!

I continued my goal-scoring form.

Against the odds, as it looked unlikely at the beginning of the year, in September, Angela and I were, thankfully, able to embark on a, pre-booked, cruise around the British Isles, in celebration of our Golden Wedding anniversary. It was a wonderful holiday and even the British weather celebrated, with us, in Mediterranean style.

On the exact date of our Anniversary, we were in the ship's theatre watching the entertainment. The compere asked the audience whether there were any couples celebrating their wedding anniversaries. There were quite a number and he then asked if there were any golden wedding couples. There were two other couples besides us. He then asked if there was anybody celebrating their Diamond Wedding. Again, there were three couples! Finally, he asked if there was anybody present who had been married longer than sixty years. One couple put their hands up. He went over to them with the microphone in his hand and asked the husband to what he attributed his long marriage.

"I couldn't stop breathing", he replied

His wife, when asked the same question, said,

"Bloody tolerance!"

When the show had ended, we stood on the deck of the ship. It was a warm, calm night. The waning crescent moon floated in a starlit sky with its reflection mirrored in a serene sea. It crossed my mind that we had been together for fifty years, and that moon, and those stars had been with us every step of the way.

When Angela and I made our vows to one another "…for richer, for poorer, in sickness and in health…" all those years ago, we were young, with our life together stretching before us. Like most young couples, we were in love, sharing a magical day with our friends and families. The promises we made to each other were certainly sincere. But we, like others, when reciting those solemn promises, would not know or have any understanding of what consequences these words could have on both our futures.

Half a century later, we were again standing side by side, but this time, reflecting on a long marriage. Yes, it was time to revisit the vows, and see how they had panned out.

Rich? We had accumulated three daughters, three sons-in-law and five grandsons. That is riches galore!

Poor? We had certainly had our moments!

Health? I believe that we have been lucky for most of our lives, and I can say, without qualification, that I've been well looked-after!

Sickness?

I guess, that by now, you would have read a bit about that!
Yes, I reckon we can safely say that we have been there, seen it,
done it and probably, if they manufacture such things, deserved
our golden tee-shirts.

The Winding Road to Recovery

"Wake up, it's 2019! Happy New Year!"

I woke Angela up from a deep sleep that the TV planners had successfully lulled her into. We opened a bottle of champagne and toasted the year to come and the old year that we had left behind.

Recovery is still ongoing, but I am fortunate to carry no visible infirmity. This is obviously a blessing but occasionally can be a cause for misunderstandings and embarrassment.

On a hot summer's day, I was walking up a steep hill and I stopped to drink from a bottle of water. I threw back my head which brought on a fit of dizziness and I had to grab hold of some adjacent railings to stop myself from falling. At that moment a couple walked by and the woman said to her partner, "Isn't it disgusting! Drunk at ten o'clock in the morning!"

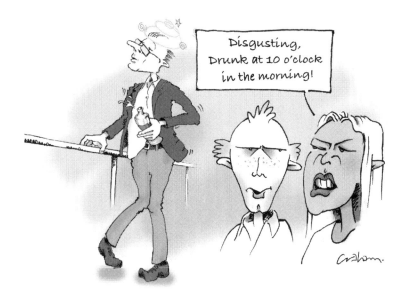

Sitting in judgement can sometimes be an imprecise preoccupation.

Thanks to the skills of the medical staff at the District Hospital, the local NHS Community Team, the support of my wife Angela, the family and the good wishes and encouragement from so many friends, my active life has been extended. I will never be able to show my gratitude enough, and it is for this reason that I have offered my services to the Stroke Association, and in my role as an Ambassador, I intend to spread the message of 'Stroke Awareness' by giving talks and arranging events within the community.

As Angela and I raised our glasses, we acknowledged that 2017 had, for me, been the year of the hat-trick, whilst 2018 had been the year for making goals, and as for 2019 and beyond, we promised ourselves, that the bucket list would be regularly topped-up and many more boxes would be ticked.

Have you been affected by Stroke?

Either as a survivor, the family or friend of a stroke survivor or as a Carer?

Like me, you will, I am sure, find the stroke Association helpful.

Any questions about stroke?

Call the stroke Association Helpline 0303 3033 100

There are a wide range of leaflets that that you might find useful.

- Understanding stroke
- The effects of Stroke
- Rehabilitation/recovery
- Life after Stroke
- Supporting a stroke survivor

All of these can be downloaded for free or printed copies can be ordered from the Stroke Association website;

www. stroke.org.uk/shop/information-leaflets

43244817R00063

Printed in Poland
by Amazon Fulfillment
Poland Sp. z o.o., Wrocław